THE
PATIENT'S
ORDEAL

Medical Ethics series

David H. Smith and
Robert M. Veatch, Editors

THE
PATIENT'S
ORDEAL

William F. May

Indiana University Press

BLOOMINGTON AND INDIANAPOLIS

First Midland Book Edition 1994

The paper used in this publication meets the minimum requirements of
American National Standard for Information Sciences—Permanence of
Paper for Printed Library Materials, ANSI Z39.48-1984.
⊗™
Manufactured in the United States of America

Library of Congress Cataloging-in-Publication Data
May, William F.
The patient's ordeal / William F. May.
p.   cm. — (Medical ethics series)
ISBN 0-253-33717-8 (alk. paper)
1. Medical ethics.   2. Patients—Psychology.   3. Decision-making
(Ethics)   4. Suffering.   I. Title.   II. Series.
R724.M285 1991
174'.2—dc20   90-45841

ISBN 0-253-20870 -x (pbk.)

2 3 4 5 6 99 98 97 96 95 94

For Lewis Soens

C O N T E N T S

ACKNOWLEDGMENTS

Like most writers in the field of medical ethics I have benefited from invitations to give lectures and papers before interdisciplinary and interprofessional groups. Such events provide the teacher with much-needed interim deadlines, the advantage of criticism, and the opportunity to write for conference proceedings early drafts of material that may eventually appear much revised in journals or books. In my case, I must acknowledge with thanks my indebtedness to the following:

Texas Tech University invited me to give a paper October 3–4, 1986, on the Dax case at a conference on "Paternalism Vs. Autonomy" in honor of Don Cowart (Dax), a severe burn victim who had graduated the previous spring from Texas Tech Law School. That essay, which appeared as "Dealing with Catastrophe" in *Dax's Case: Essays in Medical Ethics and Human Meaning*, Lonnie Kliever, editor (Dallas: Southern Methodist University Press, 1989), has undergone substantial revision and expansion for my chapter here on "The Burned."

Professor Warren Reich convened a conference on the authority of experience in medical ethics, February 11–12, 1989, at the I. H. Page Center, the Cleveland Clinic, which let me first work, under the title "From Expertise to Experience," on the links between the introduction for this volume and the first chapter, "The Burned."

As holder of the Joseph P. Kennedy, Sr. Chair in Christian Ethics at the Kennedy Institute of Ethics, Georgetown University, 1980–1985, I felt obliged to become better acquainted with the problems which the retarded and their families endure. I presented the earliest draft of my chapter on "The Retarded" at a conference at the Medical School, East Carolina University, under the title "Parenting, Bonding, and Valuing the Retarded Child," subsequently published in *Natural Abilities and Perceived Worth: Rights, Values and Retarded Persons*, Loretta Kopelman and John Moskop, editors, in the Philosophy and Medicine Series, Vol. 16 (Dordrecht, The Netherlands: D. Reidel Publishing Co., 1983).

For the opportunity to work on "The Retarded Institutionalized," I am indebted to Mary Lingerfelt-Heckrotte and Val Carmine, remarkable staff members at the Caswell Center, Kinston, North Carolina, who, in their "Inside/Out Program," let me spend a weekend with the profoundly retarded as a boarder at the Caswell Center.

A lecture for the Southern Methodist University lecture series on "Surrogate Motherhood and the Marketplace" eventually led to a short piece published under that title in *Second Opinion*, Vol. 9 (Park Ridge, Ill.: The Park Ridge Center, 1988), which I have revised and expanded for the chapter on "The Gestated and the Sold."

An invitation to address the Churchwomen United of Dallas on the subject of domestic violence eventually yielded extensive and helpful contacts with victims of battering and with professionals aiding the battered at the Family Place, Dallas, and the North Dallas Family Place HELP Center, Sherry G. Lundberg, Director.

In preparing the chapter on "The Molested," I received help from Linda Wassenich, Executive Director, Incest Recovery, Dallas, from Dr. Alayne Yates, of the Health Services Center and Department of Medicine, University of Arizona, Tucson, who granted me permission to use her taped interviews with two sisters, and from the Child Protection Services and Los Familios of that city.

The Hastings Center invited me to present my first effort on the elderly, published under the title "Who Cares for the Elderly?" in *The Hastings Center Report* (December 1982), 33–37. My chapter on "The Aged" builds on materials not only from that essay but also from "The Virtues and Vices of the Elderly," published in Great Britain in *Socio-Economic Planning Sciences*, Vol. 19, No. 4 (Pergamon Press, Ltd., 1985), pp. 255–262 and in *What Does It Mean to Grow Old? Reflections from the Humanities*, Thomas R. Cole and Sally Gadow, eds. (Durham, N. C.: Duke University Press, 1986), pp. 41–61.

Discussions with Professor Thomas F. McGovern, Department of Psychiatry, University Health Science Center, Texas Tech University, and with various professionals at the Lutheran Center for Substance Abuse, Park Ridge, Illinois, helped me in the course of developing the chapter on "The Afflicted Assisting the Afflicted: Alcoholics Anonymous." Dr. McGovern read and offered editorial suggestions on the results.

My presidential address for the American Academy of Religion eventually appeared as "Institutions as Symbols of Death" in the *Journal of the American Academy of Religion* 44:2 (June 1976), 211–223. This address served as the first draft for my chapter in this volume on "Afflicting the Afflicted: Total Institutions."

The chapter on "The Afflicted Assisting the Afflicted: Organ Transplants" has undergone the most revisions over the years. While I served as co-chair of the Research Group on Death and Dying at the Hastings Center, I presented to the Group and thereafter published "Attitudes Toward the Newly Dead; Some Implications for Organ Transplants," *Hastings Center Studies* 1:1 (1973), pp. 3–13. That essay and "Religious Justifications for Donating Body Parts," *The Hastings Center Report*, Vol.

15, No. 1 (February 1985), pp. 38–42, and "Religious Obstacles and Warrants for the Donation of Body Parts," *Transplantation Proceedings* of the International Organ Transplant Forum, Vol. 20, No. 1, Suppl. 1 (February 1988), pp. 1079–83, comprise various growth rings in the chapter that eventually appears in this volume.

Austin Presbyterian Theological Seminary of Austin, Texas invited me to deliver the Thomas White Currie Lectures at the seminary January 29–February 1, 1990. The Currie Lectures contributed to four chapters in *The Patient's Ordeal*. My thanks go to Dr. Jack L. Stotts, president of the seminary, and to innumerable other colleagues at other institutions whose invitations, encouragement, and criticisms have kept me moving on this project.

The poem "Lapis Lazuli" is reprinted with permission of Macmillan Publishing Company from the *Collected Poems of W. B. Yeats*, copyright 1940 by Georgie Yeats, renewed in 1968 by Bertha Georgie Yeats, Michael Butler Yeats, and Anne Yeats. Lines from W. H. Auden's "The Sea and the Mirror" are reprinted from *W. H. Auden: Collected Poems*, edited by Edward Mendelson, by permission of Random House, Inc.

Colleagues in my field whose own fine work keeps me reaching for the best I can do include Professor Emeritus Julian N. Hartt and Professors William Lee Miller and James Childress of the University of Virginia, Professor Stanley Hauerwas of Duke University, Dr. Daniel Callahan of the Hastings Center, Professor Leon Kass of the University of Chicago, Dr. James Wind of the Park Ridge Center, and Professor Gilbert Meilaender of Oberlin College.

At home here in Dallas, I wish to express publicly my gratitude to my patrons, Cary and Ann Maguire, gracious and public-spirited people, who endowed the Cary M. Maguire Chair in Ethics which I hold at Southern Methodist University. Their generous support across five years, including a sabbatical leave the fall of 1989, has made possible this work. A further grant from the Vidda Foundation provided me with special assistance on this book.

I have also been very fortunate in the administrative assistants who have helped me at the university, Mildred Pinkston and Susie Streng. The sociologists would call them the "underemployed," persons of talent and substance upon whom nonprofit institutions such as universities unduly depend. Their personal contributions to my work vastly exceed the managerial and processing tasks that job descriptions comprehend. In this project I am particularly grateful to Ms. Streng, who guided this manuscript patiently and intelligently through more revisions than even our computer can remember.

My editors, to whom has fallen the role of superego in this project, include Robert Veatch, Director of the Kennedy Institute of Ethics, Georgetown University, and David H. Smith, Director of the Poynter Center, Indiana University. Together, they serve as general editors of the Indiana University Press series on medical ethics. Nancy Ann Miller, editor at the Press, offered many helpful suggestions which I have only imperfectly realized in the final text.

My personal debts are unceasing to Beverly May and our four grown children, Catherine, Ted, David, and Lisa, whose sometimes amused love helped mature a father and author in ways he could not have foretold or adequately repay. But, then, family life mercifully frees one from the tit for tat of indebtedness.

And, finally, I must single out Professor Adolph Lewis Soens of the University of Notre Dame, friend, editor, and boot-camp stern reader of this manuscript, who helped make the book better than it was while courteously letting it be what it is.

THE
PATIENT'S
ORDEAL

INTRODUCTION

During the spring of 1976, I realized that I would need some clinical experience in a hospital if I were to continue writing in the field of medical ethics. The award of an Open Faculty Fellowship from the Lilly Endowment, under a program specially designed to rescue academics from the ivory tower, enabled me to spend the following year as an observer at the teaching hospital of Cornell Medical College in New York City. There, I went on rounds with attending physicians and their platoons of young residents, listened to their whispered and hurried discussions of cases in the hallways, watched surgeons scrub and then cut and burn their way through malignancies, and sensed the intramural irritations that beset any group of professionals under pressure. The year's immersion provided me with resources for writing *The Physician's Covenant*.

Some thirteen years later, however, while rereading my field notes from that year, I realized how readily I adopted the doctor's angle of vision on the hospital scene. I focused largely on the doctor's practice rather than on the patient's sense of medical crisis, on the rhythms and tempo with which professionals deliver their services rather than on the ordeals which patients suffer. My own personal focus on the doctor, moreover, largely reflected and repeated the broader preoccupation of the field of medical ethics. Moralists have concentrated chiefly on the ethics of the professional, not on the ethics of the patient and the patient's family. They have reflected more on the professional's quandaries than on the patient's ordeals.

To prepare for this book on the problems that persist long after the doctors have ordered staff to escort their patients to the hospital door, I have needed and tried to acquire a more direct acquaintance with patients and their plight. I have also had to depart from the analytical style of most writing in the field of medical ethics. I have relied instead on an approach often reportorial and interpretive rather than casuistical.

No one, of course, engages in interpretation without bringing to a subject the traditions that have formed him, which in my case, I must own, are partly literary, partly phenomenological, and partly religious; and, occasionally, I will attempt to make that religious framework explicit. I will do so not simply because a particular theological tradition has formed me but because the crises that patients face often trouble them religiously. Illness wrenches them out of their familiar world, its succor and safeties, and suspends them over a religious abyss.

This book differs from the many volumes written in the past fifteen years about medical ethics. Ethicists have flooded practitioners with elegant advice on such issues as in vitro fertilization, experimentation on human subjects, abortion, informed consent, genetic screening and counseling, and organ transplants. But they have provided less insight for practitioners and lay people about the patient's ordeal.

Insight into the patient's troubles usually comes from a very different source, not from the professional ethicist but from psychiatrists, sociologists, clinical psychologists, pastoral counselors, and their assorted popularizers among the newspaper columnists and "talking heads" on TV. The two sources of expertise do not often converge.

This moral inattentiveness to the patient and the patient's family did not always obtain. Ethicists once wrote with the intent of advising not only practitioners but their charges. The changed meaning which we have given to the traditional Roman Catholic notion of "extraordinary means" illustrates the point. Traditionally, moralists used the term "extraordinary means" to refer not simply to technical medical efforts beyond the ordinary but also to the heavy financial and emotional burdens which the patient, family members, and friends might have to endure long after the physician accomplishes his spectacular work.[1] Thus the distinction between ordinary and extraordinary traditionally helped the patient and the patient's family to recognize that they need not inevitably take on responsibilities that exceeded their resources and capacities. For example, the pious family need not invariably undertake the exceptional burden of a pilgrimage to Lourdes, the functional equivalent of a modern trek to the Mayo Clinic. The Catholic distinctions, in force today, would mercifully spare families some of the grotesque results that medical ingenuity, in tandem with the runaway power of guilt in family life, can sometimes produce.

More recently, however, the term "extraordinary means" largely serves the professional. It offers guidelines to professionals on the permissible limits of medical treatment. It suggests that the doctor need not bring down on the patient's head an avalanche of "heroic" measures to save his life. However, to equate the heroic with the aggressiveness of the doctor's technical interventions cruelly overlooks those who bear the true weight of heroism. The real burden of heroism falls not on hero-making members of the draft board who select civilians for military service but upon those civilians whom they have chosen to endure the rigors of combat. Similarly, the heavy burden of heroism in medicine falls not on the physician but on the patient and the patient's family, as they often face, after the successful rescue, an extraordinarily long and heavy responsibility of chronic care. The definition of the extraordinary should comprehend the full range of those burdens which care entails. It should not designate only the more intense but short-term aggressive measures in the intensive care unit. Such a narrow definition serves chiefly not the family but the superintending professional.

This book attempts to reactivate an earlier moral tradition: it seeks to reckon with the moral problems which the patient and the patient's family face. But in refocusing attention on those who suffer tribulation, rather than on their would-be rescuers,[2] we need to emphasize a different part of the field of ethics. Modern philosophers and theologians have concentrated chiefly on moral dilemmas. They like to identify quandaries that the decision-maker faces and then search for moral rules and principles that will help to solve or resolve these moral binds. This case-oriented view of ethics fits smoothly in the curriculum of medical schools and teaching hospitals since medical education already focuses on cases. Moralists accordingly have produced impressive work on confidentiality, truth-telling, conflict of interest, pulling the plug, and the like. But this approach does not offer much insight into the ordeals confronting patients that do not wholly admit of solution. Such problems must be faced rather than solved.

T. S. Eliot once pointed to this second range of problems.[3] At the close of a lecture on a serious issue in American life, an undergraduate arose to ask him urgently, "Mr. Eliot, what are we going to do about the problem you have discussed?" Mr. Eliot replied, in effect, "You have asked the wrong question. You must understand that we face two types of problems in life. One kind of problem provokes the question, 'What are we going to do about it?' The other kind poses the subtler question, 'How do we behave towards it?'" The first type of problem demands relatively technical, pragmatic, and tactical responses that will eliminate the difficulty; the second poses deeper challenges which no specific policy, strategy, or behavior can dissolve. The problem will persist. It requires behavior that sensitively, decorously, and appropriately fits the perduring challenge. In Gabriel Marcel's language, the latter type of problem resembles a mystery more than a puzzle; it demands a response that resembles a ritual repeated more than a technique.

Most of the deeper moral demands in life require fitting rituals rather than technical responses: the conflict between the generations, the intricacy of signals between the sexes, the mystery of birth, the health crisis, and the ordeal of fading powers and death. "I could do nothing about the death of my husband," the wife of a college president once said to me. "The chief question I faced was whether I could rise to the occasion." With one stroke, his death altered her daily life and intimacy and transformed her from a person with a clear-cut public role in the college to a superfluity. How could she rise to an occasion that redefined every moment of her daily life?

To be sure, the events of courting and love, birth, generational conflict, sickness, and death present us with something to do; but more important, they also confront us with someone to be. They assault our identity.

At one level, adolescents embody a series of complex problems for their parents to solve. But most of the turmoil occurs at deeper levels, as parents seek to cope with changes in the child's identity—and not only the child's. Parents find it difficult enough to take in their stride the profound changes which their children undergo in adolescence. But they discover, to their consternation, that the child also assaults their identity; the child redefines them as old just when they feel themselves to be at the peak of their powers. The child sees them as intrusive, awkward, out of it, an embarrassment, and not, disconcertingly enough, for anything discrete which they have done. Rather, their very existence embarrasses the child, who would prefer to believe that he or she came into the world by some mysterious act of creation out of nothing. The adolescent finds his parents' worries about him and their pride in him equally incalculable burdens; and he wishes devoutly that some tutor in the sky would teach them how to behave, which is to say, not at all like parents.

Similarly, courtship, marriage, and bearing an infant pose problems to solve, but far more profoundly they assault identity and force the self to redefine itself. Young men and women spend half their waking hours mastering social techniques, figuring out how to manage and handle the opposite sex. But they often end up with just that mate upon whom their techniques do not work. For better or for worse, they must figure out how to respond to the rhythms, tempo, and signals of the person whom they cannot manipulate, who unexpectedly has forced off balance their own inward selves.

Pregnancy and birth pose for the young mother and father a series of signs marking discrete tasks to perform and apparent crises to learn how to take in their stride. Benjamin Spock for one generation and Penelope Leach for another have written guides to help the conscientious parent. But birthing and parenting, at their deepest levels, profoundly assault and alter human identity; they limit and redefine the parents' freedom and their future; the advent of the child suddenly converts the couple's pad into a nest and reminds the parents of their own impinging mortality.

Old age also poses a series of problems, both for the elderly and for their adult children: how to supply the elderly father with transportation when his eyesight fails and his reflexes no longer respond at the wheel of the car; or how to monitor the widowed mother daily so that the inadvertent fall in the kitchen does not lead to an isolated and desperate death. In response to such practical problems, B. F. Skinner, the behaviorist, published a book offering helpful, little tricks for handling forgetfulness, impaired movement, loss of appetite, and the like. But Skinner did not address the deeper challenges that come to the elderly not simply as people who need, for example, help to walk but who also may need to live without the ability to walk. They must become more than agents managing their own problems, they must also become authors interpreting and living out the last chapter of their lives in the midst of encroaching deprivations often insoluble.

Health crises similarly confront their victims with things to do; but, far more profoundly, as such crises assault identity, they force their victims to decide who and how they will be. The successful businessman who ponders how to save his limited and valuable time puts a telephone in his Mercedes. It lets him pursue his business and care for its details even while stalled in a traffic jam. But suddenly a blood clot stalls in his coronary artery; the rescue unit pulls him out of his car and wheels him into an intensive care unit. Suddenly he finds his time even more limited than he thought. The catastrophe confronts him with problems to solve; but these problems pale before the deeper question: who and what is he now that he has suffered this explosion from within? Accustomed to commanding his world, the patient suddenly finds himself helpless in the hands of nurses down the hospital corridor; used to total obedience from his subordinates, he discovers that the very humblest of his subordinates, his own body, has rebelled against him.

The language of the surgery team reflects the profound changes the patient undergoes. Staff members regularly identify surgery patients as pre-op day one, post-op day two, or post-op day four. These designations serve the staff functionally and prosaically to flag the services scheduled for a particular day and to mark the standards for the patient's progress and recovery. Symbolically, however, the marking of the calendar can also signify a great deal more for the patient. It reflects the patient's sense of a changed and often reconceived and reordered life. Surgery and serious illness traumatize the calendar. The woman refers to "before my surgery last October" or "before my stroke last summer." The man thinks, "before my heart attack last February." The crisis divides and reorders time. It can loom, in the personal scheme of things, as large as 4 B.C. and A.D. 30 or A.D. 1990. The crisis serves as sacred event in the sense that it galvanizes time around it—before and after.

An older couple looks forward to the birth of their child. They have solved many problems. They have money in the bank, a home in the making, and a Gerber baby in the offing. But that Down's syndrome look in the nursery forces them to bury their carefully laid plans for the extension of their life through their son.

The elderly man endures irreversible changes after he retires—decreasing energy, the loosening face, the death of a mate, the howl of the wolf at 3:00 a.m. which rouses him nightly too early from sleep; and his lab workup signals yet a further problem about to surface: the hypertension that lurks symptomless within the body but could change everything with a single cerebral catastrophe. What decisions must he make? Many, to be sure. But even deeper, how can he reconstruct himself to meet daily these changes?

The doctor, the plumber, and the expert may puzzle to solve problems. Once they solve a problem, they move on to other, perhaps different, certainly new quandaries. As they handle cases, they enhance their expertise and sharpen their skills, but, traditionally conceived, they themselves do not usually change. In a sense, *qua* expert, they have little history; self-transformation is not usually at issue.

The person, however, who experiences a catastrophe moves from life through a kind of death into some sort of new identity. She participates in making history thereby. She partly shapes her own narrative in response to fateful events. In the course of that shaping, she will need to solve problems. But those problems do not pose the real issue. She herself is the problem.

The patient's experience resembles less the therapist's expertise than it does that sense of experience which W. Jackson Bate invoked in his biography of Samuel Johnson. "We are speaking of 'experience' in the vivid Latin sense as something genuinely won in the hard way—*ex periculo*, 'from danger' or 'from peril.' (From the Greek *peran* to 'pass through' and *peira*, 'trial' or 'risk'; cognates range from 'fare' in the sense of making a journey to 'pirate' and 'pilgrim.')"[4]

The German word for experience, *Erfahrung*, similarly suggests a perilous journey. A particularly difficult case may put a professional "through the ropes," as it were, subject her to a kind of ordeal, but once solved, a given problem makes no further demands on the professional, except at the technical level. The solution releases her from tension. The moral life in the professional setting is unheroic—not that it includes no agony, but that agonizing fills only a temporary phase of decision-making from which, in a given case, one expects release.

(It should be conceded that quandaries of great intensity do not remain purely technical for sensitive practitioners. In facing them, they may also acquire a history. Along with the family, they may face their own coefficient of adversity. The decision, for example, to pull the plug on the terminally ill patient poses a question about the physician's own identity. If the physician accepts the hitherto prevailing view of the medical profession as an unconditional fight against death, then pulling the plug on the patient in effect pulls the plug on himself or herself. Even to contemplate that action requires that physicians stand back from their ordinary self-perception and open themselves up to a very different view of professional purpose. To move in that direction, professionals must let themselves in for a possible change in identity hardly anticipated when they first learned to draw blood and read EKGs.)

When the medical staff has finished its work and snatched the patient from the jaws of biological death, the agony has just begun for some of the patients to whom we now turn. Thrown out into a no-man's land, with but few resources from former life, such a person faces much more than a quandary requiring a solution. In an unheroic age, she must unexpectedly push out into the unknown, where each day may pose an agony, without her own new identity in place. She may need to invent, discover, and receive, minute by minute, the person moving through a mined and stricken field.

As a way of indicating this range of problems that do not go away, I have organized this book around a series of past participles: the burned, the retarded, the battered, the molested, the aged. These conditions, and others like them, score a person deeply and often demand changes in identity. However, the use of past participles poses a danger. Society often stigmatizes and hides people under such categories, as though persons so afflicted disappear into the condition. One brother, after years of coping with inquiries about his mildly retarded brother, responded to a stranger's inquiry about him by identifying him not with his class condition among the retarded but as a self-employed business man. He had been wrong to reduce his brother to his affliction. We must, even while classifying, avoid reducing people who suffer from these various assaults on their identity to participial afflictions. Rather, we must do full justice to the moral magnitude of their response.

In choosing groups of people who face severe assaults on their identity, one also risks exaggerating the difficulties people face. Most human trouble hardly imposes ordeals as extreme as those discussed in this book. Patients going to a hospital have usually suffered neither the dramatic trauma nor the rigors of treatment which the burn patient, for example, undergoes. Does one, then, mislead by concentrating in this book not on ordinary illness but on the severities of the burn case, not on the conventional gestation of a baby but on the complexities of surrogate motherhood, not on the birth of the normal child but on the life of the retarded child, not on the average family squabbling but on the tensions surrounding the molested child and the battered spouse? Such extreme cases, however, command attention not simply because we find them dramatically compelling; the extreme case exposes clearly those challenges to identity which show only subtly and obscurely in the less dramatic medical and other crises which ordinary folk endure.

In this book, therefore, I will attend largely to extreme cases but hope to interpret them in such a way as to help illuminate what often happens in less cataclysmic illness, and, more broadly, to cast some light on some nonmedical crises. An extraordinary event draws our attention not simply because it fascinates us with an exaggerated story-line but because it also uncovers the basic terms of ordeals which we tend, to our disadvantage, to repress or ignore in ourselves.

The first case, dealing with the burn victim, but not this case alone, reminds us further that the catastrophic assault on the victim's identity includes not simply the original episode but also its debilitating biological consequences and the various ordeals that treatment imposes. In important ways, the patient may experience the treatment program itself as a sort of continuing death. Consignment to the total institution and to the rigors of treatment there often disrupts the patient's sense of his own body, rips him out of his ordinary community and identity, and disconnects him from the overarching order, rhythm, and meaning of his former life. Thus the patient often experiences the treatment of his afflictions as another, longer affliction.

The patient's experience of treatment as an ordeal hardly argues against hospitals' rigorous treatment programs, or against total institutions for the chronically and severely impaired. It suggests simply that their effectiveness may depend at least in part upon their capacity to reckon with this dimension of the patient's plight. No one, moreover, can fully understand the problems which caregivers face in persuading patients to follow a regimen, the ambivalences which patients feel toward their treatment—and the high rates of recidivism—without understanding that the reconstructed identity toward which healing must point does not loom before the patient as an unambiguously desirable goal. The reconstruction does not merely plaster something new and good and affirmative upon his old life and ways. It also threatens the patient with the loss of his former life, which—however much it may have caused his current misery—may look, retrospectively, precious. An understanding father, about to register his 170-pound adolescent boy at the fat farm for a month, delays registering him for an hour so they can go off and have a "memorial cheeseburger" together. Even rehabilitation can impose its reasons for grief.

COMMON STRUCTURAL FEATURES

The ordeals covered in this book vary considerably, and I will attempt to respect the particulars of each. But they also resemble one another. Catastrophic illness, whatever its form, confronts the patient with death, and not because the patient has nearly died, though he or she may have, but because the catastrophe attacks the patient's basic identity as a human being. Patients, moreover, experience that identity (and therefore their tribulation) in three dimensions.

Before illness, the patient identifies with her body, with her community, and with the ultimate. The self does not float free behind these identities; it does not draw its life from itself. The self is ecstatic; it pitches itself out beyond itself and identifies in all sorts of ways, wittingly and unwittingly, with these three, depending heavily and daily upon each. Whatever separates the self from these identities imposes upon the self the shudder of death.

The self identifies with its body in at least three ways. In the first instance, the body supplies the self with its means of controlling its world (feet for walking, tongue for talking, eyes for inspecting, hands for managing, muscles for exerting). Except as the self uses flesh instrumentally, it cannot master or possess its world. When illness assaults the flesh, it therefore impairs and diminishes the self's possession and control of its world and reminds the self of that final dispossession which is death. A man who has brutally exploited his body as an instrument of aggression against his world suddenly suffers a heart attack. The very flesh through which he exerted mastery falters from within. Self-confidence also collapses when the patient loses body-confidence. He flounders helplessly in the hands of others, unable to control noises down the hall that disturb his sleep. Under these circumstances, the apparatus of medicine compounds his problem. Even while ministering to him, it reminds him of his helplessness and therefore discredits all his attempts to solve the problem of his existence through mastery alone.

The body, in the second instance, serves as the site in and through which the self sees the world, disclosed in all its random glory. Through the five senses the self experiences the sun's dazzle, the city's hum, the brush of air on the skin, the mate's fragrance, and the tang of grape on the tongue. And through the sixth sense, the so-called kinesthetic sense, the self perceives its own position, movement, energy, and tension in the midst of this inflooding sense experience. The senses together also allow the self to behold the world through ritual, art, and daily routine.

Illness benumbs the senses and denies the self those incredibly varied delights which the world, unbidden, supplies the self, in the midst of its controlling routines. Nor does treatment purely and simply restore the self to its lost sensitivities. The medicine against pain dulls the senses. The sleeping pill clouds the mind. The heavy tranquilizer may succeed in halting the runaway agitation, but the patient pays a high price. He feels like a fish removed from the natural play of the water, gaffed and stunned in the bottom of the boat. The patient's isolation in the hospital further impoverishes the patient's senses: the hospital imposes upon him a functionally blank, salt-free environment, convenient for staff and treatment plans but aesthetically bare; the hospital environment lacks those singularities of sound, sight, color, taste, and smell that give shade and depth and surface to ordinary life. Patients express this self-alienating deprivation of their senses when they say they weren't their usual selves.

Finally, the body serves as the medium through which the self discloses itself to others. One does not need to be an existentialist to know that a person not only *has* a body; in a sense, she is her body. The adolescent girl, the woman in midlife, the man about to appear for his job interview, know that gesture, tone, carriage, and kinetic ease or the lack of it fatefully define the self in its commerce with others. The dynamics of such body language are, of course, complicated. The body learns how to veil itself in the course of its self-disclosure. Gestures not only signal but also, mercifully, help to obscure inner feeling. The adolescent's awkwardness partly results from his sense that his body sticks out like a sore thumb. He has not yet acquired a style—a control over his bearing—which provides him with a kind of social fig leaf. He does not yet know how to spare himself the awkwardness of instant revelation. He feels exposed, rather than revealed, and therefore always vulnerable, on the verge of shame. Nevertheless, despite these complexities and in the midst of them, the self manages to reveal itself to its neighbor in and through the living flesh.

Catastrophic illness disorients the self in its complicated veiling and unveiling through the medium of the body. The disfiguring burn, the stroke-distorted face, and the cancer-wasted body—as well as uninvited adolescent fat—alter the self's sense of itself both in its self-presentation and in its self-withholding. What the self shows no longer seems itself, and yet the self must own it. The self feels alienated from itself in its own unveiling. The body juts out and obtrudes.

Hospitalization further compounds the problem of the self's identity with its body. The patient's hospital garment, so efficiently designed and justified for the handling of personal hygiene, both conceals and exposes the body. The flapping smock both provokes and symbolizes the self's enhanced exposure to shame. The resulting blush of shame on the face similarly supplies the self with a covering but also signals the self's sense that it has lost control of its borders, its easy sovereignty, if you will, over its self-disclosure and self-withholding. Sensitive health care practitioners develop routines for acknowledging the patient's dignity in the midst of indignity, the respect owed even the bodies of the most senile and imbecilic. And funeral rites have always acknowledged that even in death the body reflects, however stiffly it masks, the person who once inhabited it.

The self also identifies with its family and community. This bonding in intimate relations goes so deep that a catastrophe that befalls the son or the daughter effectively befalls the parent. The mother who pleads with the reckless daughter, "Don't do this to me again," leaves herself open to a huge misunderstanding. The daughter takes the statement as a sign of the mother's heartless self-absorption, her inability to think of anyone but herself. In fact, the mother has so indissolubly identified with her daughter and her destiny that her daughter's self-inflicted wound also cuts the mother to the bone.

The birth of the retarded child, the fateful accident to the mate, the demented parent, these and other catastrophes can impose a kind of deep meltdown in the self which leaves it endangered. The medical literature supplies abundant evidence of the degree to which people who have experienced major "life changes" lie open and vulnerable to yet further catastrophes of their own.

Sociologists have used cooler language to describe the self's identity with its community, and the corresponding trauma which illness imposes. They have noted that the self identifies with its community partly by assuming and internalizing specific social roles. It acquires a status as mother, father, brother, daughter, computer analyst, Presbyterian, or unemployed. Not that the self entirely vanishes into these social roles. A role in the ancient theatrical sense of the term also serves as a mask that bestows upon the self a measure of privacy behind its several identities. The self stands silhouetted but also mercifully concealed behind its *personae*.

A catastrophe cuts off the victim from the several established identities that had structured his world. He enters into an *anomie*. He deteriorates from agent into patient, triply passive to the ravages of the disease, the ministrations of the professional, and the rigors of the treatment. Further, in forfeiting his social roles, he also forfeits the several layers of civilian garb that protected his privacy and dons the hospital smock which symbolizes the general immodesty of his social plight. Sickness leaves him without his usual cover. Disease now tags him as a cancer victim, a paraplegic, or an AIDS patient.

If his disease is terminal, his community of intimates may try to shield him from this knowledge. He then finds himself in an unresolved social world. On the one hand, the conspiracy of silence to which his family subjects him imposes on him a kind of premature burial. Intimates suddenly become aliens, since two important features of intimacy —an intertwined future and an ability to talk together about the future —disappear. Death wipes out the future and silence wipes out the sharing, leaving him stranded amongst aliens. On the other hand, signals do get through even in the midst of silence: the mate's tenderness, above and beyond the usual, the visiting child's conversations that steer around the future, let the patient know that he is in mortal trouble, a trouble that has altered the old inflections of intimacy. He is both buried and unburied—on the borderline, as it were—an alien amongst the living.

The self, finally, identifies with the transcendent. I do not refer here simply to the commitments which the explicitly religious person makes to an official tradition and its god, but to those connections which the self makes, whether conventionally religious or not, with those patterns and powers that go beyond, yet sustain, his life, perhaps unreflected upon, not prayed to, but that keep his life on a firm footing and that put a spring into his step.

Most people connect with the transcendent or express their "ultimate concerns" chiefly through rituals. The rituals in question include official rites; the morning prayers of Christian, Jew, or Native American can set the mode for the day. But, more broadly, rituals cover a whole range of repeated actions that conform to and represent the foundational events and the patterns of meaning in people's lives. How one rises to challenge, eats, cleanses oneself, greets one's fellows, and shuts down the day—these repeated actions signal the way in which one connects with the ultimate. These rituals are internalized as habitual structures of character that both derive from, flourish within, and, in turn, give rise to other largely repeated actions.

Modern moralists tend to miss the connection between our daily rites and moral behavior because they concentrate on special situations in which we do not know what to do. They emphasize too much those moments of puzzlement when the individual, otherwise immersed in routine, appears to be without shape and form, poised neutrally between alternatives, uncertain as to which way to jump. They deal too little with our actions when we know what to do, with those great overarching rhythms that pattern life. Moralists must reckon, to be sure, with breaks in pattern, but, if they would study life as most actually live it, they must illuminate as well habitual rituals of work, bread, love, rest, and play.

And, of course, a major illness upsets these powerful routines; it expels the patient out beyond habitual structures, familiar supports, and consolations. The patient experiences comprehensively what the sociologists term *anomie* or what the Psalmist and, later, Jesus, put more bluntly: "My God, my God, why has thou forsaken me?"

Ordeals of this magnitude pose questions at every level of the patient's being, embodied, social, and spiritual. At the least, they deepen the meaning of the so-called "hard case" in quandary ethics. Conventionally, the hard case presents us with an objective conflict between goods or evils no matter which way we turn. If we choose one good, we exclude another; if we avoid one evil, we run into another. But subjectively, the hard case confronts us with difficult going no matter which choice we make. Each path will impose on us its own coefficient of adversity.

In effect, then, most hard cases entail two decisions. First and most obvious, one must resolve the original dilemma—should one pull the plug or not, should one tell the truth or not. Second, and less obvious, one must decide and determine to make good on the decision; one must resolve to marshal the personal resources to see it through.

On the whole, "quandary ethics" emphasizes the first decision: Do I unload the bleak news? Do I let my patient die? "Virtue ethics," generally, though not exclusively, emphasizes the second decision: How do I stand by and make good on or deal with the consequences of my original choice?

In ordinary decisions we tend to emphasize the first decision. To cite a trivial illustration: A friend once called me to secure information that might help him solve a problem. Harvard, Yale, and Princeton had just accepted his child, and he wanted advice from me that would help them choose the right university for the son to attend. I responded, I must confess, somewhat impatiently. My friend knew that his son could get a superb education at any one of the three institutions. But, no matter which institution the son attended he was likely to face, as a new student from a great distance, a rough patch adjusting to his life there. The boy would far more likely survive the turbulence of the first year away from home if he himself made the choice, be the reasons for the choice ever so whimsical or arbitrary from the father's point of view. Conversely, he would less likely do well if he thought himself nudged and steered into a decision by his father's old friends. In this case, the decision to make good on the decision exceeded in importance the over-scrutinized quandary.

While emphasizing the importance of this second decision, one should neither isolate it from the original decision nor exaggerate it. The two decisions and the resources they require often interconnect. The wise resolution of the original quandary, for example, often depends upon a veritable choir of virtues: wisdom, courage, justice, self-restraint, fidelity, benevolence, honesty, and humility. Further, the subsequent determination to make good on the decision often depends upon the essential soundness of the original choice and the adroit resolution of a series of secondary issues that flow from it. Thus, the importance of the second decision should not be exaggerated. Clearly the agent's resolve does not of itself make a bad, original choice good. Pro-choicers go too far when they claim that it matters not what a person chooses as long as he chooses freely. That I have chosen a particular course of action hardly of itself makes it right. But, just as clearly, my resoluteness, or the lack of it, in carrying forward a decision can affect mightily, for good or for ill, the result; and, reflexively, my subjective irresolution can often create havoc in an otherwise unexceptionable original choice.

On the whole, medical ethics has tended to explore those moral issues that cluster around the admittedly important question "What are we going to do about it?" but at the expense of those deep, troubling issues which patients and families often face: How can they manage —whatever the decision or whatever the event—to rise to the occasion? This book deals largely with the latter question.

THE BURNED

THE EDITORS OF A BOOK on the Dax case sent me the audiovisual tape of the interview with Donald (Dax) Cowart but five months passed before I could force myself to watch it.[1] The reason for delay goes deeper than the teacher's tendency to put off writing. My own record on burn cases suggests a more troubling aversion. Fifteen years ago, while spending a sabbatical year as an observer on various hospital services, I arranged to visit the burn unit, but somehow I never made that visit. My fear, both then and now, blurts out a major problem that Dax, and all who have suffered catastrophic burns, face daily. After the surgeons have done their best and built a face they consider a technical success, the scarred patient must cope with the averted eyes of others.

Strangers stare rudely or quickly shift their eyes as they recognize the magnitude of what they have seen. Professionals at work in the crisis centers—nurses, social workers, and other therapists—burn out after six months or so. Acquaintances and colleagues gradually manage to stabilize their behavior but the victim's plight still sends a deep tremor through their lives. Meanwhile, family members and friends fixate on an event that has irrevocably altered a portion of themselves.

But the deepest aversion besets the victim himself. He knows that his very existence now repels others; they recoil first, and only later talk, listen, and venture a smile. His helplessness in the midst of these shocks produces a second generation of responses less innocent than the first. The foolish inspire his contempt; the nervous, his impatience;

the transient philanthropists and tourists, his anger; and friends and professionals, the temptation to manipulate. No sensitive patient can fail to note his own unsavory responses. Thus he experiences a profound aversion not only to the catastrophe that has befallen him but also to himself. Neither the technical successes of medicine nor the company of others can ease his problem. In leaving him disfigured, medicine leaves him with a chronic sorrow, a limitless grief, which the aversive swoon of others salutes but cannot heal.

Dax himself goes to the heart of the event in an interview eleven years after the explosion and fire that killed his father and severely burned two thirds of his own body, including his face, his eyes, his ears, his hands, and his feet, leaving charred flesh and scorched bone where, an instant before, a 27-year-old man had walked freely. This young, recently discharged jet pilot and veteran of Viet Nam had excelled as a golfer, surfer, football player, runner, and rodeo cowboy. Like many other burn victims, he remained wholly conscious during the disaster. He thought, while plunging through three walls of fire, rolling on the ground, and running again, "It couldn't be happening—a dream, a nightmare—but it really was happening." The first man on the scene, a farmer, exclaimed, "O my God!" and Donald Cowart said, "Go help my father," and then asked the farmer for a gun: "Don't you see, I am a dead man. I can't live."

That horrific statement goes to the heart of his problem. He does not predict "I will die." Medical experts, who would lift his untouchable body by his belt, take him to the hospital, and eventually conclude there, "No, we can keep you alive," could prove his prediction wrong. He states, rather, "I am [already] a dead man." Whatever that dreadful statement means, it flatly distinguishes human life from mere biological persistence. (Don Cowart, after all, still persisted when he called Donald Cowart dead.) Human death does not terminate a biological organism alone.

Don Cowart's laconic self-appraisal exposes the shallowness of all efforts to interpret catastrophe by appeal to the notion of "quality of life." He knows that the fires have not merely scorched his quality of life, shadowed the margins of his life; the explosion has immolated him. The Don Cowart that was has died.

After the explosion, Donald Cowart eventually changes his name to Dax. He does so partly for a functional reason. Despite the ingenuity of reconstructive surgery, he will never be able to write his full name again; he can manage only Dax. But the name change also fits symbolically. He knows that Donald Cowart has, if not biologically, existentially died; he must assume a new identity.

This experience of burning as death includes not only the flames but also the series of convulsive impacts the body subsequently undergoes, the ordeal of medical treatment, and the scarred results of that treatment. Death turns out to be not one concluded and conclusive event but a detailed, continuous, enforced and reinforced condition.

Instant Impairment of Function. The fire burned off one eye completely, two-thirds of his skin, his eyelids, the flesh of his face, and his ears instantly. Unlike other burn victims, he did not breathe in smoke and fire, which would have seared his lungs and blocked his breathing. He did not suffer brain damage or the loss of consciousness (though in the ensuing treatment, he experiences what the literature refers to as psychotic breaks, as he hallucinates and imagines the worst of the nursing staff). We can assume that he could still smell and taste (though what he smells, burned tissue and, ultimately, infection, will offend him and others). He loses most of both hands, he cannot at that point walk, he cannot bear touching and being touched.

These various losses, quite apart from the complexities and pain of future treatment, will blast that bodily identity upon which each of us depends to master some portion of the world, through the hands, feet, eyes, and tongue. Dax's losses are particularly great since he has fallen from such a great height. The explosion and fire destroy Don Cowart the fighter pilot and athlete.

Such losses also dam, at least temporarily, the sluice gate of the senses. Nurse Leslie E. Einfeldt of the University of Washington Burn Center reports more generally about the severely burned patient: "All five of his senses have not only been overwhelmingly assaulted but have been rendered temporarily inoperative."[2]

The Assault of Treatment. The original blast persists, in effect, in the efforts to treat and heal in the intensive care unit of the Burn Center. Just two examples of the effort to treat—intubating and tubbing—suffice to illustrate the power of that assault.

The average 154-pound man requires a daily fluid intake of 3 liters to compensate for the body's normal fluid losses through urine, sweat, and breathing. The unassaulted body needs no more liquid since it enjoys a delicate homeostasis, a splendid harmony, which the skin preserves by clothing the body. The skin armors the body against the world: it keeps the precious within and the noxious without; it prevents fragile protoplasm from oozing into the surroundings and bars invading microorganisms. It regulates temperature and fluid loss, and keeps in balance deeper body functions. Pimply in youth, wrinkled in age, the skin defines our extended selves, our health, and our limits.[3]

The person burned through the skin suffers a rude shock to this integral functioning. The durable elastic barrier that holds precious fluids within, through which he experiences the pleasures of his universe, and which keeps poison and decomposition at bay, burns away. Without the skin to prevent evaporation, the body loses massive amounts of fluids. The body reacts by descending into the deep physiological shock of hypovolemia. Cell walls destroyed, the body starts to ooze plasma. The burned body may need not 3 but 14 liters of fluid in the first 24 hours following a 50-percent, third-degree burn. Somehow the body must cope with this depletion just as the burn accelerates the victim's metabolic rate, further increasing his need for food.

The shock of the initial widespread breach of the body's surface extends itself inward, forcing successive waves of collapse, compromising further walls, protective mechanisms, and body functions. Specifically, the shock produces tiny sores in the gastrointestinal tract with some sloughing of the gastric mucosa. These sores paralyze the intestinal tract; the victim cannot process food. Not only does the world about him recoil, but his own digestive system profoundly recoils and balks. The patient may also experience a kind of psychological equivalent of this intestinal recoil with the onset of depression and anorexia.

To keep the burned body alive, doctors use intravenous feeding, unloading massive amounts of fluid into the leaking tank of the body in an effort to nourish and protect other organs and to keep the body from drying up. IV feeding, however, also endangers; the fluids swell the already bloated points of entry and overload kidneys that cannot handle as much fluid as they could before the burn. The general swelling blocks circulation, and that in turn hampers healing and threatens to destroy surviving, less damaged skin. The medical staff, in brief, balances destruction and pain of one kind against destruction and pain of another, and the patient suffers therapies that maintain life, but attack each other.

Tubbing, Pain, and Cold. The medical staff must fight bacterial invasion and infections (since the loss of skin has weakened the immune systems) by cleansing wounds, cutting away dead or contaminated tissue (debridement), removing scales, handling other dying tissues by enzymatic removal, and repeatedly applying salves to the wounds and changing bandages. In addition to these painful procedures, the staff subjects the patient to daily tubbings. Immersion in a Hubbard tank helps prevent infection and removes old water-soluble, cream-based dressings and dead skin and crusts. Daily tubbing also eases joint motion and thus helps the patient save some abilities that let him act rather than suffer. During the procedure, the staff keeps the room temperature at 80 degrees Fahrenheit and the water temperature in the tank at 98.5 to 100 degrees. The patient, however, shivers, since the body, robbed of its natural clothing, cannot regulate its own temperature. Meanwhile, staff members work at room temperatures much too hot for their own comfort. They inflict cold on a shivering patient while they themselves are uncomfortably warm.

The accident originally imposed upon the patient a baptism by fire;

now tubbing imposes a daily and frightful baptism by water. It causes pain so excruciating that one surgeon advised hospital architects to move the tank room away from the burn unit so as to keep the patient's bed a respite from the place of torture and, in a phrase that speaks volumes, to avoid "sensitizing the other patients."[4]

This is not to say that the burn victim escapes pain away from the tubbing room. Partial-thickness burns release pain-causing prostaglandins and histamines around the burned area. Exposure to the air causes pain. Heterotopic bone forming in the joints hurts, and stretching shriveled contractures also hurts. The burn victim continues to hurt even after his wounds heal; in this respect, he resembles the arthritic patient who aches at every change in the weather. All strategies to dull pain, whether by hypnosis, acupuncture, or drugs, also have their limits. While the pain caused by partial-thickness burns will respond to non-opiate prostaglandin inhibitors, the pain resulting from full-thickness burns in the course of tubbing treatment responds only partly to opiate analgesics. Fortunately, improvements in treatment since the early seventies have lessened somewhat the physical pain that a patient in Dax's condition would likely suffer, though the residual pain is still formidable.

Perhaps more than any other feature of illness, pain forces the patient into *anomie*; it tears him out of the ordinary patterns and rhythms of his life. Those patterns give meaning and purpose to his life, partly immediate and partly ultimate. Pain disconnects. It makes the body, which we largely take for granted in the pursuit of ends, suddenly obtrude and distract from our goals, as it recoils protectively from, or writhes in the midst of, pain. The toothache, the throbbing headache, nausea, the scorched body—these pains take over; they isolate us from community and they disorient us from ends. Disease and pain, in the jargon of one author, are "telic dysfunctional." They decentralize the "higher *telos* of the organism, and [cause] its loss of dominance over the lower tele,"[5] a state which Jesus expressed more starkly with his cry of abandonment from the cross.

Disfigurement. None of the ordeals of treatment, however, compares with the final deprivation, the psychic wound of mutilation. The surgeons concede that, while they can partially restore function, in many cases they can do much less to restore appearance. The language of the experts sometimes retreats into euphemism. A surgeon's sensitive essay on disfigurement hides under the stilted title "The Limitations of Aesthetic Reconstruction." The editors of the volume *Comprehensive Approaches to the Burned Person* discreetly tuck away this chapter at the end of the book, but the limitations of the medical arts break out starkly in sentence after sentence in this and other essays: ". . . the ultimate or final reconstruction of the severely burned face can be expected to remain, if not positively repellent and grotesque, at least unsatisfactory and unpleasing."[6] Or again, "The surgeon must accept that what delights him as a technical result may still be a horror to his patient."[7] And, most poignantly, "Our work requires putting a new facial garment, often a garment of sorrow, on these patients."[8]

The surgeon, Dr. Constable, chooses his metaphor carefully. The word "rehabilitation," in its Latin root, *habil*, means to clothe. The soul, in a sense, never exposes itself utterly naked. It presents itself to another in and through the body, the soul's clothing, the medium that veils and unveils it. In their first hope, family members bring to the surgeon earlier pictures of the burned victim to guide in the restoration. But, whatever rehabilitation does, it does not restore. Not that the surgeon's art lacks ingenuity. But even at best, making full use of skin grafts, synthetic coverings, and pressure garments to flatten the thick scar tissue and to soften its lines, the surgeon cannot, on the severely burned face, restore looks. That term, "look," is not an abstract object of aesthetic judgment. It is always *someone's* look and therefore presents and forms the self. The burn patient discovers that an alien has now taken over that presentation. A casement has replaced the soul's own clothing. Hence, the burned child sometimes finds himself teased and called a "mummy."

While armored in scar tissue, the victim feels wholly vulnerable and therefore ashamed. The look of his face flies out ahead of him, beyond his control. He cannot hope for the good luck to interact spontaneously with others. His disfigurement stiffens in advance their response. Thus the scar not only encases and distorts the victim; it also encases and distorts the responses of others, a predicament which they solve by avoidance. Nancy Hansen, a physical therapist, reports that the problem of reentering society preoccupied a group of adolescent burn patients more than any other consequence of their accident.[9] Dax commented eleven years after his injuries, "Because of my disfigurement, I wondered whether I would ever have a meaningful relationship with the opposite sex. I considered not going out in public at all. Finally, I had such a bad case of cabin fever, I said, to hell with it. Though it was easier for me because I couldn't see. It would be harder for somebody who wasn't blind."[10]

LIFE VS. QUALITY OF LIFE

At first glance, Dax's case seems to fit conventional controversy in medical ethics. Most moral issues in medicine today turn on the conflicts between two rival values—life vs. quality of life—and between two rival principles for determining the decision-maker—paternalism vs. autonomy. Pro-lifers exalt life as the absolute good and oppose any and all decisions to terminate life regardless of life's quality. Dax, on the other hand, appears to join those who invoke quality of life, as he pleads with his mother and his managers to allow him to die.

This substantive dispute between the values of life and quality of life quickly leads to a controversy over who should decide. Dax's doctors and the medical establishment tend to fight unconditionally for life. Therefore, Dax must contest their right to decide whether he lives or dies. He invokes the principle of autonomy, asserts his right of self-determination, and inveighs against the preemptive and paternalistic action of the medical staff.

The Dax case, however, challenges this conventional analysis of the great moral issues in medical ethics. When we see the basic issue in medical catastrophe as a conflict between the values of life and quality of life, we make a series of false assumptions. First, we think of life as unilinear. We imagine it a straight line that begins with birth and concludes with biological death. The line has a beginning and an end. All else in between we characterize by the substantive: life. The line changes, of course. The living creature undergoes, through his own making and through fate and fortune, a series of modifications for which we reserve the term "quality of life." Sometimes the line fattens and we think of the subject's quality of life as good; at other times it thins out and we characterize the quality of life as poor. A varying quality of life simply suggests variations in the same substantive—life. It allows for qualifications or modifications, but no more.

The current formulation of the arguments between pro-lifers and pro-quality-of-lifers tends to obscure and distort the plight of Dax and others who have suffered a major illness or trauma. The traumatized person has not experienced his life as a continuous straight line that will eventually end in biological death. He perceives the catastrophe as annihilating. The lifeline has already broken, whether through a single event, a series of events, or a single event that sets off a series of secondary and devastating consequences, including the ordeal of treatment. The highway accident, the devastating fire, the mental breakdown of a family member, the irreversible, progressive and immobilizing disease, or the nasty divorce; they do not merely qualify life at its edges. They break off the old life.

Those who originally advanced the term "quality of life" hoped by that emphasis to prevent an exclusive concentration on biological life alone. They believed that decision-makers must take into account changes in life's quality. But the term "quality of life," with its notion of measurable changes, positive and negative, on a continuum, tells us too little about actual experience. The patient must deal not with a continuous line that thickens and thins, depending upon circumstances, but with a substantive break and a new line.

The burn patient faces, then, an existential problem that the arith-metical quandary of life vs. quality of life cannot describe: how does one respond to one's death or the threat of one's death? to a piercing, sun-blackening, oxygen-removing, flesh-charring, chilling, stilling, numbing, isolating death? If the patient revives after such events, he must reconstruct afresh, tap new power, and appropriate patterns that help define a new existence. One cannot talk simply of a new accessory here, a change of venue there, but—as one image puts it—of a new Phoenix that must emerge from the ashes.

A conceptual difficulty emerges in the Dax case. Can we call the charred victim "dead," in the state we are describing? When Dax says "I am a dead man," does not the "I" live to say "I am dead"? Does he not use "death," metaphorically and melodramatically, rather than realistically, to describe his state and condition? How can one talk about the destruction of an essence when the substance still persists under the name Dax? Does not common sense tell us to relegate any and all changes experienced along the way to qualifications of life, and no more?

The conceptual difficulty recedes in this case if we recognize that human existence is ecstatic in the sense that the biological line alone does not define it. The individual largely lives in that which lies beyond him. He tries to secure his existence, to be sure, in and through the capacities, powers, and assets he thinks he can dispose, but living pitches him out beyond himself into the world that he savors, the several communities to which he attaches himself, and, above all else, to those patterns and powers that surround him with meaning and establish the rhythm, tempo, and round of his daily life. Strip him of these and he suffers a fundamental break in his existence that besets him with death.

Unfortunately, therapists can only tinker with the details of things —we can get the patient a typewriter that he can work with his teeth, or braces that will help him stand up; or we can do another series of operations that will retrieve some thumb-finger opposition in his hand; or we can simulate some eyebrows for him—all these technical accom-plishments, proffered by the surgeon and varied therapists, will signifi-cantly improve the patient's quality of life, but they will not revive, they will only embitter him in their triviality if he himself has not mourned and buried an old identity and moved toward a new self on the other side of the ashes. Only then can he take and accept and find any cause for celebration in this or that trinket that medical ingenuity can offer.

Death, Perilous Passage, and Rebirth. Is there any precedent for this very different interpretation of the patient's problem that breaks with the one-dimensional linearity of Western medicine and Western society as a whole? In my judgment, a much older tradition of healing, based on a very different sense of human existence, supplies the more adequate alternative. Traditional societies, if we follow Van Gennep and Van der Leeuw,[11] did not view life as a straight line, bounded on one side by birth and on the far side by death. Rather, death (and birth) intersected the line throughout.

Periodically, men and women in traditional societies died to life as it was. They had to doff their identities, suffer a perilous period of transition, unclothed, until they entered into a new life, defined by a new identity, new patterns, and accession to new power. "Birth, naming, initiation, marriage, sickness and recovery, the start and end of a long journey, the outbreak of war and conclusion of peace, death and burial are all points of contact between Power and life."[12] One interprets such points inadequately as mere events. Contact with supernal power required celebration, but not in our trivializing, modern sense of that term. Such contacts require rites that bury the past, rites that carry the subject safely through a period of acute vulnerability, and rites of incorporation into a new estate. Not only traditional societies but also Christian communities use the language of death and resurrection to emphasize the sharpness of the break between the old and the new. The metaphor of undressing and dressing expresses both ceremonially and substantively the alterations demanded as the soul puts off the old and puts on the new.

We see vestigial remains of such altering events in, for example, the crowning of a sovereign or the monk's undertaking of his final vows. Queen Elizabeth, on the occasion of her coronation, symbolically disrobed, signaling that she must put her old, private identity behind her as she accepts her new, royal estate. Shakespeare's *Henry IV*, Part II emphasizes the tragic consequences of this kind of abrupt change, as the newly crowned King Henry repudiates his old, drunken crony, Falstaff.

> I know thee not, old man. Fall to the prayers.
> How ill white hairs become a fool and jester!
> . . . .
> Reply not to me with a fool-born jest.
> Presume not that I am the thing I was,
> For God doth know, so shall the world perceive,
> That I have turned away from my former self.
> So will I those that kept me company.[13]

Similarly, the monk who prostrates himself on the floor to take final vows acknowledges symbolically the end to his old life and the birth of a new.

The burns that we have described in this essay destroy the soul's clothing and leave the frail self in naked agony. Then, God willing, the soul begins to grow a new self. The surgeon may be competent to graft skin, but his skill alone will not avail to reclothe the soul.

The interpretation herein offered of burn patients applies more broadly to the victims of various catastrophes. The man who suffers a major heart attack, the woman who bears a retarded child, the subject of a biopsy that announces an invasive tumor—all these victims suffer an upheaval, with or without rites, that disrupts daily rhythms, dashes hopes, and revises their sense of themselves and their past. That upheaval calls for rites of passage and a new life.

However, we had best not oversimplify or exaggerate the change. The Dax case, on which we focus here, tends to emphasize total annihilation. Short of suffering brain damage, perhaps no patient undergoes the massive alteration in self-perception and prospects that the burn victim must fear. And yet, even the burn victim and victims of other, lesser catastrophes do not suffer a total wipe-out. The image of the Phoenix, risen from the ashes, partly misleads us, because the Phoenix remembers nothing of its former life. The burn victim, however, remembers his past. The persistence of memory both establishes continuity with his past but also reinforces his sense of distance from it. He remembers what he has lost and therefore grieves more deeply. But at the same time, other elements of his former life carry over. Long-neglected assets, some strengths of character, tics of temperament, old nightmares, recurrent dreams, familiar habits of mind, and even more familiar vices may still persist. Rebirth, renewal, and reconstruction do not take place *ex nihilo*.

Not even the religious tradition that attests most radically to the theme of death and rebirth demands that one interpret this new birth as a total displacement. As the New Testament scholar and professor Wayne Meeks has noted, "the Christians could speak of dying and rising with Christ, as a second birth. . . . The radicality of the metaphors bespeaks a real experience of sharp displacement which many of the converts must have felt. [Nevertheless] . . . one cannot efface or replace the primary socialization."[14] In a sense, the change of name from Saul to Paul changes only one letter.

The complication of these continuities in the midst of discontinuity does not compromise the basic pattern of life / death / rebirth. While some elements from one's former life persist,[15] the organizing center, the referent for all else, changes. What previously occupied the margins of experience as a barely noticed incident, a spontaneous pleasure, or a casual exception to habit now looms large as a resource in one's new existence. What was marginal, episodic, contrary, and repressed before the change now begins to shape the reconstituted person. Continuity shatters; and yet fragments of the old self persist in the reconstituted self.[16]

(What, however, of the person who has already undergone a profound life change that leads to a new identity but who then suffers a
catastrophe of the magnitude of Dax's? Does he perforce submit to another destruction of identity that obliterates the recently acquired one
and assume yet a further new identity? The specific case of Christian
identity poses this question which, of course, moves beyond the particulars of the Dax case. The person who, prior to suffering a catastrophe,
has become a Christian has already submitted to an initiatory rite of
baptism, which, taken seriously, calls for a kind of Hubbard tank of
the spirit. It asks for the dying to the old man and the birth of a new
person. When, at length, this person suffers a catastrophe, does this
event perforce impose the forfeit of his faith, as he moves perilously
across the wilderness to a newly constituted self? Clearly forfeits of nom-
inal faith occur repeatedly. Faith flourishes while life runs smoothly,
the job pays well, and the cholesterol counts reassure, but it vanishes
under the crushing weight of disease, accident, market downturn, or
the loss of a child or mate. The very real possibility of such forfeit leads
Scripture to question: "When the Son of man comes, will he find faith
on earth?" (Luke 18:8)

But how do we interpret what happens to a second Christian who
has similarly suffered catastrophe but whose faith, in this instance, does
not melt down and evaporate? Somehow his new identity persists in
the midst, and in spite, of the ordeal. The burn, the heart attack, the
stroke, or the growing cancer has not utterly devoured him. His original
identity holds and endures. In this case, must we say that the categories
of death, perilous passage, and rebirth no longer apply?

The New Testament is remarkably clear in its answer to this question. It does not promise any easily persisting identity in the midst
of ordeal. The New Testament variously refers to faith as tried, tested,
proved, and tempted. These various words serve to translate the Greek
word *peirazo*, the very same term to which Samuel Johnson referred
as providing the root for our rather pale word in English, "experience,"
and the more bracing words "peril," "pirate," and "pilgrim."

Christian identity does not spare the pilgrim ordeals that test faith.
Indeed, the specific ordeal of fire breaks into the scriptural discussion
of peril: ". . . the genuineness of your faith, more precious than gold
which though perishable is tested by fire . . ." (I Peter 1:7). Or again,
"Beloved, do not be surprised at the fiery ordeal which comes upon
you to prove you, as though something strange were happening to you"
(I Peter 4:12). The latter passage, urging the Christian not to be surprised, verges on the comic. Clearly, a catastrophe batters the victim
with the experience of the strange and the estranging. It rips him out
of his familiar identity with body, community, and God and expels him
out into unfamiliar terrain. He travels confusedly as an alien in a foreign

land and feels self-alienated, disconnected, confounded, his identity imperiled. Any recovery of his religious identity will of necessity strike with the force and astonishment of rebirth. And yet, at the same time, he should not be astonished. The identity into which he is reinserted, reborn, conjoins him to the savior who himself journeyed into the far country, who himself and "in every respect has been tempted as we are" (Hebrews 4:15), who suffered an ordeal that threatened the loss of identity with body, community, and God, and who yet remains faithfully himself, the servant of God, throughout.[17] Rediscovering such a savior is not a new birth, a different birth, but a rebirth in an identity to which heretofore he perhaps only too nominally and shallowly belonged.)

Shifting the terms of discussion from life vs. quality of life to life / death / rebirth illuminates a number of issues in health care and health care ethics.

1) The choice of terms used determines the resolution of the traditional quandary as to whether one should allow the patient to die. The conventional formulation of the debate—life vs. quality of life—slants the argument in favor of the pro-lifers. The term "quality of life," while invented to focus more attention on the question of life's quality, does not fully express the deadly impact of such an accident on the core self. "Quality of life" implies that even a major burn affects only the circumstances and surfaces of life, the accidents of the self, rather than its substance. Such language predisposes one to use elaborate means to continue life under any and all circumstances. This predisposition largely rules the medical profession. The profession has tended to define itself as engaged in an unconditional fight against biological death. It does not admit the continuing death that it sometimes imposes on the patient. In the worst of burn cases, the patient faces two catastrophes: first, his original burn; second, the catastrophe of survival imposed by medicine, a catastrophe which the term "diminished quality of life" only partly reflects.

2) As it tilts the debate in favor of life, the vocabulary that pits life against quality of life slights the importance of providing follow-up resources to support the patient after the medical crisis. Because that support affects only life's quality, society provides massively for acute care but only grudgingly for rehabilitative and chronic care. We have developed, of course, post-crisis therapies to rehabilitate the patient, but the spreadsheets show we put our big money into emergency, acute, and intensive treatment, not into rehabilitative and chronic care.

3) This neglect of rehabilitation may in the long run weaken society's support for the original medical decision to enforce survival. While the community provides massively for acute care, it feels free at the outset to relegate questions of life's quality to the individual. Some pro-

lifers believe that the community has done its job once it has behaved like a gang of deputies, saved a victim's biological life, but then ridden off, leaving the survivor stranded. This pro-life callousness, however, eventually provokes a moral and political revulsion which undermines the commitment to life as a good. (This revulsion unfortunately does not appreciate the important moral differences between two distinct parties in the pro-life movement: one pro-life group supports life for nine months and then condemns the mother and abandons the child; another group admits the importance of helping the child, once born, and the mother.)

The linked terms "life / death / rebirth" make it clear that the responsibility of the community has just begun if it has imposed survival upon the individual in the midst of what the individual in some circumstances can only experience as a fearful ordeal.

4) Concretely, the vocabulary of rebirth and reconstruction requires the community to increase investment in rehabilitative and chronic care. This vocabulary would emphasize as relevant interventionists not only medical staff but also other healers, such as nurses, social workers, physical therapists, occupational therapists, pastors, chaplains, and other patients who have survived similar ordeals. The emergency and survival treatments of the surgeon and the physician prevent biological death but do not begin to touch the problems that biological life now imposes upon the patient and the patient's family. Technique and treatment supply means to accomplish ends; but the patient faces a crisis in the ends themselves. Other health care practitioners, pastors, family members, and the patients who have crossed the same terrain may help the patient more than practitioners of merely technical skill. These less glamorous figures loom larger to the degree that our language highlights the task of reconstruction and rebirth.

5) This emphasis on the language of reconstruction and rebirth also forces one to recognize that the chief figure in the cast of characters is neither the surgeon nor other health care practitioners but the patient. Thrown out into a no-man's land, often without much help from his former life, cut off from his former goals, his old skills suddenly irrelevant, aspirations unattainable, old identity and enthusiasms on the ash heap, the old skin unwearable, and the familiar rhythms and tempo of life faltering, such a person faces vastly more than a quandary soluble through the technical assistance of others. And even when therapists can offer substantive help about ends, goals, purposes, and meaning, such help avails little unless the patient actively participates in the enterprise. The patient occupies the central position as the decision-maker, since he must variously confirm and live with the consequences of the original decision to keep him alive.

6) Emphasis on the language of rebirth and upon the patient as the primary figure in the narrative does not eliminate the traditional

problem of paternalism in medicine, however. Indeed, one might argue that the language of death and rebirth intensifies the problem. If a patient merely suffers a change in the quality of his life, then one can assume substantial continuity between his two estates. But if one talks about an alteration in substance, then one might argue that the confounded patient cannot make judgments about a possible new identity and estate. He cannot engage in his self-creation. He needs experienced decision-makers acting for him in the absence of a newly established center for his being. Thus the Dax case and many lesser catastrophes continue to pose the question as to who makes the final and fateful decisions.

PATERNALISM VS. AUTONOMY

An appeal to the metaphor of parenting to interpret the healer's work does not automatically set off the ethical alarm bells in me as it does in the antipaternalists. While the parental analogy does not offer the best metaphor for understanding the healing art, it helps. The healer should, like a good parent, show compassion for the patient's plight and a readiness to sacrifice for the patient's good. Like the parental, the therapeutic relationship presupposes a marked imbalance in knowledge and power which, unchecked by compassion and self-giving, can quickly deteriorate into indifference or rank exploitation.

When Dax's caregivers refused to heed his wishes to let him die, he accused them of paternalism. Paternalism changes the parental metaphor into an ideology. Paternalism justifies unilateral interference, manipulation, or bypassing the freedom of another adult on the ground that the authority knows that this intrusion will best serve the patient's welfare.

Paternalists usually justify their unilateral decisions to intervene on one or more of four grounds:[18] (1) the patient lacks the mental competence—either temporarily or permanently—to absorb, understand, or act on information relevant to his case; (2) the imposed limit on the patient's freedom to decide is relatively trivial; (3) only the proposed limitation can protect the patient from a substantial harm; or (4) the imposed limit will produce a substantial good. By using these arguments, the physician implicitly concedes that he or she must justify the limiting intervention. Theoretically, the patient need not justify his rejection of treatment.

Clearly the staff in the Dax case could not defend paternalistic interventions on the second ground, that they imposed only trivial limits on the patient. The staff flatly refused to grant Dax's petition to let him die—hardly a trivial interdiction of his wishes—and imposed on him a long series of draconian measures—mostly against his wishes—all of them causing him anything but trivial pain.

The third argument—protection against an evil—probably figures most often in the set of reasons parents give themselves for limiting their children's freedom, and physicians, their patients' autonomy. Anxiety comes with parenting. One wants to take those whom one loves out of harm's way. Since, moreover, the wayward freedom of one's children so often leads them to injury, the parent hopes to prevent harm by preemptively limiting freedom. Or, alternatively, parents recognize that their gloomy knowledge may dispirit and crush their children, hence they limit freedom rather than explain danger. Parents love anxiously. Thus they build an imprisoning sanctuary around their children.

The medical staff similarly seeks to protect patients from the evil of death. Hence a paternalistic staff must limit the patient's wayward freedom and inexpert knowledge, both of which hinder an effective fight against death. The staff justifies managing and manipulating the patient in order to stave off the ultimate destroyer. Paternalistic love justifies a manipulative strategy for the battle.

While this third consideration often governs the surgical team in the acute phase of the crisis, the fourth argument chiefly attracts the therapists who take over after the crisis—the nurse, the social worker, perhaps the psychiatrist, and the chaplain. The fight against death draws to a close and the problems associated with the reconstruction of life rise now to head the agenda. The post-crisis staff intends to promote a good rather than merely prevent an evil. Since reconstructing life requires some measure of cooperation from the patient, the crude, overt paternalism—or, more inclusively, parentalism—of the crisis team fades. To the degree that paternalism survives, it survives in velvet, more managerial, gloves. Professionals pride themselves on their expertise, their skill and cunning, in steering their charges toward the preferred shore.

I use the word "steering" advisedly. Clearly treatment requires, especially in the case of a burn victim, a steadfast dedication to the regimen. The fight against death continues in the midst of efforts to reconstruct life. Halting, even for a short time, the changes in bandages and ointments, the tubbing, and the splinting of the patient does not simply delay recovery, it increases destruction. Such a halt converts second-degree into third-degree burns; it increases the need for autografts using skin materials already in tragically short supply; it cripples and immobilizes the patient. The patient, incapacitated by pain and drugs, cannot steer the craft. "Leave the driving to us," so the argument goes. (The medical community wants the patient to collaborate in accepting the delivery of technical services, but these technical services may assault the patient as pure torture without collaboration at a deeper level, which may be possible only as the patient has begun to move inwardly beyond an old and toward a new identity.)

The first argument for paternalistic intervention—the impaired autonomy of the patient—shapes the Dax case; it overlaps and intertwines with the generally fixed commitment of the medical profession to fight against the evil of death. Professionals working in burn units do not need much encouragement to act on what they perceive to be the patient's massively impaired capacity to decide. At the outset, the victim of a severe accident suffers post-trauma depression. He lacks, in the judgment of the professional, general psychological competence. The professional has seen too many post-trauma depressives who have demanded that physicians stop treating them and then changed their minds later. But this suspicion of post-traumatic depressives discredits the patient's wishes and casts a long shadow into the future, particularly when the patient's opposition to a procedure seems to prove the patient's impaired capacity. The burden of proof thus effectively shifts from the physician having to justify his paternalistic intervention to the patient having to prove his competence. The videotapes on the Dax case portray a patient forced to prove his sanity in order to break out of the trap.

Burn unit professionals can also point to unrelenting external burdens associated with treatment and a horribly insulted nervous system as grounds for denying the patient's competence. This assessment brands the patient not quite as psychotic, but as sufficiently impaired to lack ability to identify and steer his life toward his own best interests.

Finally, the paternalist can argue that the patient—whatever his emotional state—lacks knowledge that would let him appreciate the evils that the treatment may prevent or the goods it may promote. The patient's life, after all, has not merely changed; the catastrophe has often destroyed the very substance of that life. The patient has entered into a no-man's land, or, at least, a land into which few have ventured. The patient cannot know what lies ahead. Therefore he cannot decide competently.

Of course, in an important sense, the doctors know less about this forbidding country ahead than does the patient. The doctors have not themselves gone directly through the experience of death, a perilous interim, and rebirth, and, even if they had, they would not know altogether what the experience would mean existentially to this particular patient.

But the doctors do know what surface, technical reconstruction they can achieve, and they have watched other patients travel along roughly the same path. Thus they urge the patient to go along with the therapy. They say, in effect, "Persist in the treatment plan. Don't ask us to allow you to die now. Let us finish our work. Then see what you've got, what life is yours. Make at that point a more informed choice." In effect, the doctors apply the old adage "Don't show a fool a half-finished piece of work." The shortsighted inspect the dismantled car or the construction site when things are torn up and assume that's the way they will always be. The surgeon thus appeals, in this case, not to an argument based on his professional commitment to life nor to the patient's future quality of life but rather to the eventual quality of the patient's decision. "Wait and see what we have produced and what you yourself have become. Your decision then will be better informed." Moreover, "Once we have provided you with some substitute thumb / finger opposition, if you still want to die you can kill yourself. You won't have to ask us to do it."[19]

But Dax remains unmoved. He states he cannot stand the price he would have to pay to improve the quality of that decision. He does not want knowledge at any price. The pain is palpable and intolerable. "Please let me die." (This last response explains why Dax to this day sees no contradiction in two admissions: first, he confesses that he is glad to be alive, but, second, he still feels that his doctors wronged him by keeping him alive. If a similar catastrophe befell him now, he knows that he would not want to suffer that same magnitude of pain again. He would appeal once again: "Please let me die.")

Paternalists in family life or medicine chiefly commit the sins of the overbearing. Their sins are those of excess; they would do too much. In the midst of catastrophe, they keenly feel the absence of divine providence and substitute themselves as a minor league providence. The providence they offer does not reckon fully with the turmoil of freedom within and the pain of suffering without. In order to protect the patient, this substitute providence often withholds knowledge, subverts his freedom, and imposes one set of evils in seeking to circumvent another. Paternalists control too tightly, foist too suffocating a love on their charges. The patient, angered that this substitute providence is reducing him to the physician's property, cries, "Whose Life Is It Anyway?"[20]

Paternalism has generated a vehement opposition in our time which flies under the banner of the pro-choice movement. The term "pro-choice" covers a wide variety of positions. Some pro-choicers merely rename the quality-of-life argument. They want to *free* patients to decide on the basis of their own estimate of their life's quality. For these pro-choicers, happiness in abundance ranks as the preeminent good, and pain the preeminent evil. They want to leave the patient free to exit if, in his judgment, he chooses to escape his suffering.

In its least attractive version, the term "pro-choice" smacks a little of the marketplace. Consumers freely compare and contrast the relative quality of cars, beers, suits, dresses, houses, and lives, choosing some, rejecting others. An uncritical relativism lurks behind this version of the pro-choice position. All moral judgments merely express one's own personal preferences. *No one has the right* to interfere, advise, or judge another's choices since the ground on which one would base such interventions would itself but express an arbitrary preference.

This reduction of judgment to a mere preference, however, creates a philosophical awkwardness. It undercuts the axioms underlying all moral judgments and therefore makes it impossible to sustain the judgment that "no one has the right to interfere." The denial of right itself crumbles into mere personal taste. The appeal to a moral universal in the claim "No one has the right. . ." loses all grounding. The "pro" in pro-choice merely expresses a preference. It effervesces rather than articulates morally. Even the most consumerist of societies cannot survive without some further discussion about the reasons for the "pro" and the actual content of those choices, pro or con. Buying a plug may be a consumerist choice; pulling the plug is not.

A second pro-choice position affirms liberty as more than the expression of a mere preference; liberty itself is the necessary precondition of moral community. One cannot act morally while coerced. This position does not claim that the mere fact of my choosing freely makes any and all choices right; I must always respect the similar liberty of others. The principle of mutual respect expresses more than personal preference; it helps articulate the content of the moral community for which the principle of liberty supplies the form.

A popular version of this pro-choice position, however, ends up today generating only minimal duties. One must chiefly refrain from interfering with the liberty of others. The doctor must expertly inform the patient about the likely consequences of a treatment. But the decision about the treatment rests with the patient. This libertarian pro-choice position converts all decisions and goods (other than respect for the liberty of others) to questions of personal preference and taste. It leads to a minimalist understanding of both the state's and the professional's responsibilities. While deferring to liberty, it downplays rather too many vicious uses of liberty in our time, particularly the sins of neglect and omission.

When antipaternalism moves in this direction, it falls into a vice opposite that of the paternalists. Paternalists fall easily into the sins of the overbearing. For the sake of the patient's well-being, they override his freedom; they do too much. Antipaternalists, however, often lapse into the opposing sins of the underbearing. In reducing the professionals to mere technicians, they may do too little. They replace the paternalist's sins of commission with the minimalist's sins of omission. Now indifference and neglect replace a suffocating love. (At one level, of course, Dax's paternalists may have fallen into some of the selfsame sins of omission. While they paternalistically insisted on continuing treatment, they may have identified that treatment with largely technical services which perpetuated the horror without dealing with his real problem, the problem that he felt he had existentially died and that neither he nor the purveyor of technical services could begin to reconstruct his life.)

Pro-choice, at a third level, may affirm the moral insight anticipated in the introduction to this book. Many serious choices in life actually consist of two decisions. First, one faces an obvious quandary—for example, should one or should one not marry a specific person? Second, one faces the less obvious, but often just as important, decision to make good on the first decision. This second decision often can sustain or undo the apparently more serious original choice. The will to make good on a decision does not itself make the decision right. But irresolution can unravel the best of decisions. This insight inclines many counselors to the pro-choice position. Perhaps such counselors criticize insufficiently the actual content of decisions but, for good reason, they respect the importance of choosing determinedly in the moral life.

This resoluteness counts for a good deal in facing the harsh consequences of so-called hard cases. Out of respect for the burdens that sometimes follow in the train of a medical decision, the Catholic Church, as noted earlier, distinguished between ordinary and extraordinary means. This distinction guided not only physicians mobilizing technical resources, but also patients and families estimating the burdens they might face. The distinction respected the zone of discretionary power belonging to patients and families in deciding whether to take up extraordinary burdens, financial or otherwise. The pro-choice movement, at least in part, has wanted to save this traditional power for patients and families.

Dax's caregivers face a quandary they can quickly resolve because they can keep him alive, but he must live with the results of their decision—the extraordinary pain which his treatment entails and his suffering, for who knows how long, until his biological death. In all this, his life must reconstruct from the grave up. Paternalists do not want to grant him the power to decide whether to accept treatment; they fear that he will opt out of life. Perhaps, however, leaving the door open to the possibility of his refusing treatment may make it easier for him to accept treatment and to persevere in the consequences of that acceptance and make good. The patient's feeling that someone has slammed a door shut increases his sense of nightmare; masters who only perpetuate his misery have trapped and boxed him in. Were the door ajar, he might find it a little easier to stay in the room of pain.

The decisive defect of the paternalist position shows up in some of the literature on the burn patient. In an article on comprehensive approaches to the burned person, for example, A. Napier Baker meticulously interprets the work of the burn team in familial and parentalist metaphors. The total staff forms the "burn center family." The burn center director presides as patriarch, the head nurse as matriarch, the nurse in charge as the elder sister, and assorted other members of staff as siblings, aunts, uncles, and cousins. The author identifies the patient as the newly arrived baby. In effect, Baker's account of introducing the patient into the burn unit family elaborately parodies rebirth.

> The burned person enters into the family having experienced severe trauma. The major insult to his system and person leaves him in a state of forced dependency. He is introduced to his new family through the painfully cleansing experience of the Hubbard tank. It is as though the first changing of his diaper were marked by repeated pin sticks.[21]

The author likens members of the burned person's biological family to fiancées, to outsiders, whom the burn unit family tests in various ways before granting membership. Baker does not invoke the parental analogy merely to emphasize the dreadful physical dependency that the disaster imposes. He then tracks the patient through the various stages of growth—the defiance of the toddler, the demands and bargaining associated with toilet training, the childish demand for attention at bedtime ("why don't they ever burn their bell fingers?" one staff member moans who serves as the author's illustration of negative parenting), and the turbulences of adolescence. Finally, the patient graduates from the burn unit, that is, he "goes off to college."

The paternalist ideology misleads us if we seek to interpret through its lens the relation between the health care team and those patients who have suffered major loss. Parents have acquired their authority over their children because they have already endured in their own time what the infant / child / adolescent goes through. They have already suffered what must come to all, one way or another, in the course of their maturation.

(When children reach adolescence, they begin to contest their parents' authority not because they are fully experienced but because they believe that the world has dramatically changed since their parents acquired their views. Strictly speaking, they believe, their parents do not know what they are "going through." In any event, whether accepted or contested, parental authority rests in large part on that personal experience that freights their love.)

By this standard, professionals, on the other hand, have not endured what their patients have suffered. The patient's experience differs from the professional's expertise. Professionals do acquire the authority of a specific kind of experience, in addition to their technical expertise, but it is the experience of interventionists proximate to an event, not of its principal, however compassionately they may support the principal.

Older, more experienced members of the health care team may reasonably adopt a benignly paternalistic attitude toward new, inexperienced members of the *health care team* itself, but *not* toward the burn victim. The accident, originally, and the horrifying treatment, subsequently, resemble not at all an ordinary process of maturation, least of all the way that team members themselves have matured. Rather, the double catastrophe pushes the patient out into the terrain of the extraordinary—into an extraordinary deprivation, an intense and mercilessly regimented pain, and social hurdles that would send most team members themselves into stunned retreat. Whatever the team can do for the victim, it cannot bring him to new life without his consent. It cannot provide him with such parenting. The domestic analogy is wrong.

The patient, for better or worse, resembles not the balky toddler in the bosom of the family, but rather the agonist in Greek tragedy or the stricken religious figure cut off from the safeties of family and city. I cite these analogies not in order to flatter the patient, but simply in order to locate him. He bears the mark of the uncanny, the German term for which is the *Unheimlich*, literally, the one "not at home," the alien, the one driven out beyond the ordinary precincts of hearth and city gates, where no one in his right mind would want to venture, and who therefore sends a shudder through the rest of the community.

One may criticize such a person (one ought not to blink at his faults), but one cannot rightly patronize him. Should he choose to live, he cannot choose simply to take up his old life. He must become a new man. Don Cowart becomes Dax. No parentalist can force him down that road. No mere medical technician ever does enough to assist him along that road. To travel into that darkness requires an interior transformation, it requires ethics at the deepest level, not trivial problem-solving, but the reordering of one's identity from the ground up. The community can and must assist in countless ways. But without consent to transformation the patient cannot move from saying "please let me die" to "I am glad to be alive." That heroic movement does not vindicate his doctors, because the deeper decision must be his, and only as it is his do we see in him not simply a patient encased and obscured by the surgeon's art but the uncanny radiance of a man.

THE RETARDED

OFFSPRING OF THE lower primates cling to the bodies of their mothers; marsupials hang on for dear life. But the human infant is unable to cling. The mother must hang onto as well as carry her young. This dependency upon the mother for the simple act of carrying, the precondition of so much else, makes the human infant rely heavily on bonding. A mother must actively cradle her child, cherish it, for it to flourish.

Bonding engenders loyalty to the being and well-being of another. In a sense, "loyalty" is too weak a term. It suggests a relation that depends upon the will of both parties. Bonding describes the way in which two people settle into one another's bone marrow and kidneys, imagination and bowels. Bonding does not demand a mystical merger of identity between two partners; but it establishes a tie so powerful that neither can undertake much without reckoning with the consequences for the being and well-being of the other.

Most attempts to identify the value of the retarded child neglect the process of parenting and bonding. Aspiring to abstraction, they proceed along lines implied in the title of a conference, "Natural Abilities and Perceived Worth." They impersonally consider measurable properties (such as intelligence) that distinguish the retarded and others from zebras, parsnips, and rocks. By "abstraction" I mean the kind of assessment of natural abilities that a professional or policy-maker might make in a hospital, a prison, or a high school, an assessment cleanly distanced from a relation to the carrier of those capacities. From this lofty perspective, parental belief in worth may seem merely subjective, lacking in validity and valency.

This chapter explores, alternatively, the kind of valuing that goes on in the relation of parenting and bonding. It emphasizes a relational rather than a possessional view of the self. It explores the relationship *between* human beings for its clues to their being and value and our obligations to them, rather than assigning values according to the numbers scored. It looks to the dynamics of bonding between parents and their retarded child rather than to a distanced consideration of capacities possessed and performance attained.

Since no moral life can dodge adversity, this narrative about bonding will also have to deal with the great obstacles to bonding—both external and institutional, and internal and personal—which the parents of the retarded confront. While the parents of the retarded must overcome or circumvent these obstacles at their most difficult, such obstacles throw their shadows across all parenting, whatever the abilities of the child.

EXTERNAL OBSTACLES TO PARENTING

Most researchers have emphasized the obstacles institutions place in the way of early parenting and bonding, especially in the crucial hours and days immediately following birth. The modern nuclear family, we hear endlessly, suffers simultaneously from the absence of those community supports of family and friends that helped parents bond to their children in traditional societies and from the overbearing presence of the hospital and the medical staff at birth.

The celebrative atmosphere of home birth in traditional societies boosted the mother's growing attachment to the child. The excitement of other participants in the event aroused buoyancy and confidence in her. By contrast, the industrialized West has tended until recently to treat birth (even normal birth) "as an illness or an operation," and isolated it in an institution that often intimidates women.[1] The modern medical concern to prevent infection curtailed the physical contact between mother and child so crucial to bonding. Most normal births in the hospital condemned mothers and babies to several days of isolation and deprivation. As late as 1970, only 30 percent of mothers were permitted to touch their babies in the first days of life.

Hospitals have handled premature and abnormal babies even more antiseptically. These babies became "monstrous" in the literal sense of that term; that is, they became objects to see and point at but not to touch. Fittingly, the first director of a nursery for premature babies in this country, Martin Cooney, exhibited them at most major fairs and exhibitions in the United States from 1902 to 1940. Receipts from his *Kinderbrutanstalt* at the Chicago World's Fair of 1932 ranked second only to ticket sales for fan dancer Sally Rand—someone else to see and point at but not touch. Cooney discovered, not surprisingly, that some of the mothers whose babies he sent out on exhibition did not want them back when, as they reached five pounds, he returned them. They had not bonded. Cooney's procedures, developed in the nursery of commerce, significantly shaped methods of newborn care in the United States—and not for premature babies only.

Recent critics have severely criticized medical professionals and institutions for disrupting bonding. Some of these critics have perhaps exaggerated. They gravely assumed that actions in the first few hours and days after birth irreversibly stamp the relationship of parents to their child. They have earnestly promised almost magical results from laying the baby across the mother's warm abdomen immediately after birth. Still, these critics have a point. Klaus and Kennell report that when early mother-child cuddling is lacking, breast-feeding fails more often, child-battering increases, and some statistical differences in I.Q. and language attainment show up as much as two years later.[2]

The additional care the retarded or handicapped baby needs compounds the problem. Increased professional and institutional interventions reduce the mother's contact with the baby during the sensitive period crucial to bonding. Psychologically, the mother and father need this contact. Every mother needs time to adjust to the appearance of her infant (often one to three days); the stark information that the child suffers from something wrong heightens fears. Often seeing and touching the child—even a deformed or retarded child—make it easier for parents to cope.

Changes in hospital practices since 1970 reflect a greater institutional respect for the parents' and babies' needs to touch and bond. Although aggressive medicine still dominates the intensive care unit for children, hospitals have shown more appreciation recently for the parents' needs to know and touch and to do the handling, nurturing, and sheltering their child needs. Professionals cannot neglect these activities and treat the child simply as a bundle of medical problems—containing so many grams of body weight, lab values, and deficits—and expect the child to come home to easy and natural parental embraces.

INTERNAL OBSTACLES TO PARENTING

Probably the external, institutional obstacles to parenting and bonding would not loom so large if parents did not face even more formidable internal obstacles to bonding with their child. Parental emotions hinder bonding, whatever the institutional setting and whatever the child's status. The infant confronts its parents as a stranger, threatens to restrict their freedom, and makes them anxious about the future. The retarded child pushes each of these emotions to its extreme.

1) Moral reflection that does not reckon with the experience of the child as a stranger misses the test that individuals face in parenting and bonding. Our deepest psychic responses make us distrust and reject the stranger. This aversion showed on the day of our birth when we complained loudly about being ejected from the familiar comfort and warmth of the womb into a strange world. It appeared at seven months of age when we began to fear strangers and abandonment.[3] It continued at four years when we shied back behind our mother's skirts, as strangers leaned over, grinning, to tell us what a fine little boy or girl we were. And at ten we heard mysterious warnings not to go anywhere with strangers—strangers are tricky. Mother invested the stranger with an unspecified power to harm. Nor does adult life leave this aversion behind. Especially in this country, a country of immigrants, wave upon wave of strangers have made their way into established cities, neighborhoods, schools, unions, clubs, and businesses, assaulting the psyche and provoking patterns of recoil and aversion.

This disturbing experience of the strange stirs no less at the arrival of the newborn. In a sense, birth, especially first birth, confronts a young woman and man with the ultimate stranger, the newcomer, the absolute immigrant into this world. The young woman in *How Green Was My Valley* announces her pregnancy to her former boyfriend by saying, "We're going to have a little stranger." Something quintessentially new, and thus threatening, is coming into the world. The ceremonies of birth today, in an unfamiliar setting filled with masked officiants, reinforce the feeling of trepidation before the strange.

But the alien newcomer itself, more than the rites through which it arrives, unsettles the parents. How so? The human imagination contributes to the shock of alienation. In anticipation of their child's birth, parents tend to imagine greeting and holding a strapping, healthy baby, lustrous, smiling, and cooing at maternal care. They have already seen dozens of infants in supermarket strollers, or Gerber portraits of infants wrapped around jars on food shelves, or babies in Polaroid pictures, plump and fully human. This imaginative anticipation reduces the child-to-be to the familiar and manageable. The child will merely perpetuate, extend, and amplify the familiar world rather than push its parents into the novel and strange. The world-to-be will not shock or surprise. The present will overtake the future by way of peaceful annexation.

But the baby's arrival upsets the daydream. The mother discovers that the infant isn't herself cloned; it doesn't even resemble the father.

She has borne a prune, a monkey, a strange looking thing. Further, it imposes its strange movements, its jarring demands, its noises at all hours; it turns one's life around rather than adds something to it. When it cries one wants to mother it, and yet it also makes the stomach nervously coil.

If the ordinary child intrudes itself as a stranger, the retarded child invades. It shatters all parental expectations. It converts the daydream into a nightmare. It presents the parents with a reality so alien to all their original hopes that the event confronts them with the force of death. The arrival of the retarded child kills the dream child and forces parents to grieve its loss.[4] This grief presents them with special difficulties in attaching themselves to the actual child, since we bond—to use the jargon of experts in the field—"monotropically." Close attachments form best to one child at a time. We cannot easily bond while mourning another. "We have noted in many parents who have lost one of a twin pair that they have found it difficult to mourn completely the baby who died and at the same time to feel attached to the survivor."[5] The death of the dream child ends the world that the mother and father trusted. They can only grudgingly embrace the new world that presents itself in the real child. Not all parents of retarded infants discover immediately that their child is retarded. Sometimes they bond to the child first and only subsequently discover mild to severe retardation. Such delayed recognition, however, does not wholly eliminate the trauma of coping as the newly discovered alien appears beneath the already accepted face.

In bonding and valuing the retarded, parents must first accept strangeness and overcome the aversion strangeness entails. The Enlightenment notion of the unity of humankind, which assumes universally shared characteristics, common properties, offers little help in reckoning with the strange. The Enlightenment, idealizing tolerance and benevolence, attempted to trivialize differences by measuring them on a scale of capacities and standards. It underestimated the stranger, who upsets my universe not because he differs from me in measurable ways but because, by existing, he shatters my rules and scales. The stranger creates a hemorrhage in my universe.

We do not bond, then, in a cozy assimilation or mystical merging of two beings. Like the love that precedes them (heterosexual love means, literally, love of the strange sex), parenting, bonding, and valuing require openness to the strange, learning devotion to the other set in strangeness. Nor does healthy bonding eliminate strangeness. Martin Buber observed that "othering" goes on in the I-Thou relationship. A relationship pales and dissolves when two beings take one another wholly for granted or presume too much on likeness. They no longer need to watch, listen, or attend to one another. Strangeness is the bracer in love. From the perspective of the biblical tradition, faith warrants openness to the stranger, not by the humane and liberal assertion that we must tolerate all men because, underneath, they are all alike, but because God himself, the primordial stranger, bonds to his creatures despite the abyss between them. Theologically, we must bond because of, not despite, strangeness.

2) Parenting requires not only coping with the strange, but also losing a portion of one's freedom. Grief over the loss of freedom used to center in the institution of marriage itself. Today, however, both husband and wife work, allowing each to continue as part-time bachelors.

Having a child, more than marriage, makes the difference. Parents lose not only money (double salary), but time. The mother feels drawn to love the child, to care for it, to delight in it, but it also ties her down, takes her time. The baby turns out not to be a toy—it eats; it sleeps (at the beginning, 14 to 18 hours per day); it eliminates (at the outset, it urinates 18 times a day, defecates 4 to 7 times a day, and takes at least 8 diaper changes).

Parenting, in brief, poses the moral / metaphysical problem that *Huckleberry Finn* faced. The novel darkly suggests that love and freedom don't mix. Huck Finn runs away from his stifling hometown to freedom on the river. But, on the river, Huck meets up with Jim and bonds to him. His feeling for Jim makes him uneasy; it ties him down. Twain presents a gloomy vision; love and freedom diminish one another. Today, young people get out of the house and become sexually active and it tastes like freedom, but this freedom one day produces the event that suddenly and relentlessly ties them down. The growing bonds of love seem like bondage.

The retarded child intensifies this loss, certainly for those who keep the child home. Parenting inevitably curtails liberty, but ordinarily parents can view this loss as temporary. When their children grow up, parents hope to regain the freedom they have lost. But the retarded child does not fully grow up. Only the death of the parents—or the child—will end their responsibilities. Unless mildly retarded, the child can never take over full responsibility for his life; and he requires a much heavier investment of his parents' time in training. The retarded child's acquisition of those skills that other parents note in their children with some measure of gratification and relief—eating, dressing, personal hygiene, the mastery of social etiquette and rules governing work and play—slows down to 2/2 time. The parents either adjust their own tempo accordingly or discover family life operating on two very different beats. Either way, spontaneity and freedom in family life diminish.

3) Parenting expresses hope, but also stirs up anxiety about the future. Clearly, giving birth affirms the future. From the ancient Manichaeans forward, pessimists have always resisted bearing children. The Manichaeans loathed the material world, the body, sex, and the perpetuation of that world through progeny. The trappings of their mythology

have withered, but the basic links between pessimism about the future and a great reluctance to have children still persist to this day: "the world is already overcrowded"; "I wouldn't want to go through that again"; "it would be wrong to bring children into the world."

A willingness to bear children shows optimism, but bearing a child also stirs up anxiety about what lies ahead. The affirmation contained in a child forces parents to scout the unknown on behalf of the precious but powerless. In ordinary parenting, apprehension about the future subsides as parents immerse themselves in daily demands and joys. But fear of the future always looms over the parents of the retarded. In the first stage, parents often suspect something, they know not what. (We fear most intensely, argued the existentialists, the evil not yet revealed.) When physicians name the problem, they give it some specificity, but ordinarily do not spell out its full ramifications. As the dreadful implications and complications of the original diagnosis unfold, parents begin to generalize about the future: whatever it is, it will be bad. Therefore, defensively, they turn to the present and do what they can, one day at a time. Sufficient unto the day is the evil thereof.

Nevertheless, the long-range future still disturbs. The severely impaired child tends to be the last child in a family. Its birth tends to have a contraceptive effect. The future also looks bleak at those moments when parents see retarded adults. As much as they feel that they have come to accept their retarded child and their own responsibilities, they discover that they cannot yet accept the adolescent and the adult-to-be. Helen Featherstone describes a visit to see older children. It posed for her as a parent all over again the confrontation with the strange. "The children had lost their otherworldly charm; they were now simply psychotic adolescents. The hopes of parents and teachers had faded along with their baby fat."[6] But even if one accepts the future adult-to-be, the bleak circumstances which that adult will face cannot help but disconcert. "Most of us, for all our hopes and dreams, are still fattening up our children for the inevitable institutional kill."[7]

MOMENTS IN BONDING

Bonding is a two-way street; parents and children interact. Although we can, at present, describe only crudely the experience of bonding from the baby's point of view, we can nevertheless see that the baby that self-confidently attaches itself to its mother is likely to behave in ways that arouse more affectionate and spontaneous maternal responses. Conversely, a child who has suffered traumatic institutional separation from its mother will react with anger, anxious possessiveness, or self-protective detachment. This obstructive behavior, in turn, produces negative responses from the mother that increase the child's anger, possessive clinging, or guarded apathy.[8] Further, the varying degrees of mental retardation, from profound to mild, make a difference in the obstacles parents face in bonding. A full treatment of bonding would have to take account of these differences.

Recent efforts to describe bonding with the retarded child sound very much like Kübler-Ross on death and dying; the sequence of anger, fear, denial, bargaining, and acceptance surfaces in the discussion. This approach has the advantage of letting the actual emotions of parents into the open. As in other crises to which her stages have been applied, however, one wonders whether Kübler-Ross and those who follow her interpret these stages as descriptive or normative, chronological or concurrent, elective or compulsory.

An alternative scheme for interpreting bonding focuses less on specific emotional attitudes than on the magnitude of birth and the changes it calls for in parents' lives. Bearing a retarded child imposes upon parents an experience that corresponds structurally to those great turning points (and associated rites of passage) in traditional societies that transported people from one stage of life to another—birth, puberty, marriage, and death. The discussion of the Dax case makes it clear that these turning points included three "moments" or elements: (1) a break from the past; (2) a turbulent period of transition; and (3) entry into a new life and estate.[9] Whatever parenting a retarded child may entail emotionally for parents—fear, loneliness, resentment, and the like—it includes these three "moments." It wrenches them out of their former life, its assumptions and priorities; it produces a period of disorientation, confusion, and provisional adjustment; and, it is hoped, it ends in the parents' final attachment both to the child and to the circumstances that life with that child entails. In these respects, parenting resembles ancient rites of induction into the sacred. However, in the absence today of the definitive social rites that in traditional societies shaped and limited great crises and turning points, these "moments" do not follow in a tidy sequence. They overlap in the course of a profound sea change in the life and prospects of the parents.

Detachment from the Past. Detachment, at times, seems too mild a word; destruction more accurately tells the truth of the matter. The birth of a retarded child shatters one's world. "The world crumbled and fell around us," reports the mother of a Down's syndrome child.[10] "In one cataclysmic moment, our world had been shattered," another mother testifies.[11] Helen Featherstone, who has gathered evidence and also writes out of personal experience, states, "The shock of disability seems to obliterate the life that exists," and "threatens to define an ominous pattern for the new one."[12]

Trying to cope with the alien emphasizes this break with one's previous life. Routines, demands upon oneself and others, daily and long-range prospects change. The retarded child changes one's definitions of the important and the unimportant. The child alienates in that it estranges parents from their familiar world. Things look different—in the way parents view not only their own lives, but also the lives of their friends. Parents testify to their sense of isolation. This isolation shows up practically, but it also marks a deeper cultural isolation.

Practically, isolation begins in the hospital, where medical intervention often separates the mother not only from the child but from other mothers. It spreads as friends and relatives mumble or blurt in acknowledging the birth. (One mother reports that nothing unnerved her so much as her own mother's insistence that she institutionalize her child. Irony abounds in the advice the grandmother offered. She was attempting to mother her own daughter—to protect her from suffering. But the daughter found the advice troubling. It undermined her own ability to mother her retarded child. Her capacity to mother her child grew from the mothering she had received in childhood. But now her own mother seemed to say: "If you had been retarded, I would not have mothered you." The daughter kept her child but it disturbed other bonds.)

In time, the retarded child's special needs for care necessarily affect the family's daily routine and social life. Such needs not only throw out of balance parental efforts to give their several children equal attention, they also place early demands upon the other children as care-givers. Brothers and sisters sometimes feel cut off from their peers by their heavier responsibilities. The parent less engrossed in care also can grow to resent the special attention the retarded or the handicapped child receives. Not only is the child different, but the child's existence makes the marriage different. The primary caregiver, meanwhile, cannot help but compare her own plight (usually "her"—the world hasn't changed that much) with the lighter burdens of her contemporaries. One mother testifies that unhappiness alienates not only because others shun the unhappy but because the unhappy resent the others' happiness—especially when the fortunate take their happiness for granted.

Culturally, the birth of a retarded child cashiers not only the parents' social life but also their assumptions about prized American values: the American reliance on the wizardry of medicine, its orientation to youth as a symbol of promise, and its abhorrence of dependency. Americans have traditionally celebrated a technological triumphalism by assuming that all human problems will eventually yield to the organized assault of research and the strategic weapons generated by American research. But the parents quickly discover that medical research and the experts who wield the technologies which flow from it quickly reach their limits in helping a retarded child. A medical army marches in circles around their own tiny baby and its fateful problem. The physician cannot function heroically, but merely carries bad news. Medical magic that prolongs their child's life or patches up its other physical difficulties merely highlights medicine's inability to touch the fundamental cause of the parents' grief.

Further, the event heretically denies the conventional American attitude toward youth. As an immigrant people, Americans orient themselves more obsessively toward their children's performance than do members of more settled societies. In America, W. H. Auden once remarked, immigrant children live under the pressure to outstrip, in Great Britain, merely to live up to their parents.[13] The retarded child, however, cannot meet either demand. The child's severe impairment both shatters and yet fails to anesthetize them against the myths about youth. Parents suffer the discrepancy between myth and performance by feeling guilty for the child's shortfall. The American middle-class myth of producing the perfect child has always confused the process of manufacturing with giving birth. Americans take credit for the child as a product rather than rejoicing in it as a gift. In this atmosphere, the arrival of a retarded child signifies a personal failure rather than an imperfect gift. The child excommunicates its parents from the ordinary circle of nursery achievement. A child becomes "a dispiriting symbol of shared failure"[14] between husband and wife. The guilt and self-doubt compound the problem of attachment. As long as the child symbolizes failure, parents find it hard to love, hard to attach to, because in accepting the child, parents must ultimately learn to accept their discredited selves.

In yet another way, parents of the retarded feel isolated from the prevailing culture. Americans prize independence, both in their national and in their personal life. As a sinister obverse, they abhor dependency. Americans do not like to depend upon anyone personally and withdraw from those who threaten to depend, in turn, upon them. Europeans often complain that Americans, beneath their easy amiability, have little capacity for abiding friendship. Whether or not independence deserves praise, the failure to achieve it, either as a family or in any of its members, stigmatizes and isolates the family from others. The irremediable dependency of their severely or profoundly retarded child throws the family into a social plight that most others abhor and shun.

In a variety of ways, the retarded child disconnects its family from the culture at large. It is un-American; it makes aliens of parents, brothers, and sisters. For better or for worse, they cannot participate immediately in the technological momentum, the orientation to youth, and the pride in independence that mark their peers. They become estranged in their own culture. Loyalty to this child requires a reconsidered relation to much else.

The parents and children suffer some of the pangs of detachment from their former life even when they choose to institutionalize the retarded child, though the form of their suffering differs. In this case, the child does not obtrude daily as a stranger in the home; rather, it belongs to a strange world, a specialized world of those similarly afflicted. Part of the task of accepting the child requires accepting the strange world to which it belongs. The parents reacquire some of their lost freedom by putting the child in an institution, but feelings of guilt and ambivalence often shadow that decision. Freedom does not come as a reward for the completion of the extended training tasks which parents customarily assume, but from deputizing others to discharge parental duties. In an important sense, parents affirm the future growth of their child by institutionalizing. The institution, after all, has resources for training beyond the reach and command of the nuclear family. But, at the same time, the decision to institutionalize requires parents to recognize the definitive outer limits to the child's potential. Hope loses its euphoria. Parents suffer at the same time an experience of loss resembling the original death which the discovery of retardation imposed. Bonding originally required the burial of the dream child and now institutionalization threatens with the burial of the actual child. However right the decision to institutionalize—and it can be very right indeed—the family faces with that decision its own subsequent coefficient of adversity.

Transition. In traditional societies, many perils accompany the passage from one estate to another (birth, puberty, marriage, war, peace, death). Such a passage often entails a suspension of ordinary activities associated with the old life. A potentially confusing period, it requires specialists (priest, warrior, shaman) to supervise and assist people through the transition rites associated with the great turning points in life.

Isolation and confusion can engulf parents with the arrival of the retarded infant. Professionals can err in opposite ways in handling this difficult transition. Out of compassion, caution, or their own aversion to pain, they may unduly prolong the transition by withholding the worst news. They dole it out to the parents in bits and pieces. Sometimes such compassion misses the mark. In the absence of candor, parents often generate worse fears. Anxiety feeds on uncertainty. Indeed, the transition period cannot end if parents fear that the future may hold even worse perils not yet revealed.

At the other extreme, professionals may fail to respect sufficiently the need for a transition. They may be unduly impatient with parents and unwilling to give adequate time to let parents assimilate bad news. They assume that parents should absorb the news and get on with the program. They do not realize that this kind of news both shocks and burns its way slowly into the mind. One doctor confesses, "It isn't okay to break the news, and support them for a week, and then give them an infant stimulation program and everything is fine. Some parents turn around very fast, and some turn around slowly. . . ."[15]

Parents usually need time to reorient themselves. Freud sensed the need for this time in any profound reconstruction of the self. When asked why the analyst could not simply tell the patient the truth about himself and be done with it, Freud remarked that the truth so delivered would sit like a parallel deposit in the mind, unassimilated.[16] Just so, parents of the retarded need to assimilate. They need some time to absorb the news that severs them from their former expectations, myths, and gratifications. They also need some time to enter into their new estate. The child (and their life with the child) carries its values, but its values strike with a force that transvalues rather than merely adds to the values which the parents already profess.

The specialists required in the period of transition include more than the obstetrician or the pediatrician whose repertoire of skills hardly begins to address the problems the child and the family face. The social worker, the nurse, the physical therapist, the special educator, the rabbi, minister, or priest, and other parents who have faced similar ordeals have important roles to play. The very recital of this list reminds us that our health care system and its schedule of rewards inadequately honor those who figure large in a successful transition. Our third-party payment system rewards substantially those whose interventions hand to the parents their problem, but it provides much less adequate support to those who can give parents a helping hand with their problem. This disproportionate emphasis on acute care reduces too often the family's alternatives in care either to the expensive total institution or to the family's own limited, isolated resources. The system underfinances those supplementary services that might help make family care more tolerable and sustainable.

To assist a family wisely and enduringly, these various specialists must also help the family enlarge its sense of its own competence and resources. Eventually the family will need to review its positive assets. Such an inventory is difficult to undertake since the initial grief which the event provokes carries with it its own dark perception of the family's plight, a perception which impresses the grief-stricken as realistic. The serious accident along the highway or the discovery of the accident in one's genes both turns the world chilly and lowers one's sense of self-esteem. The victim suffers the double assault of despair and shame. Chaplains and other counselors have their work cut out for them. Admittedly, the lowering of self-esteem makes little rational sense (the self is not at fault), but, psychologically, the blow that exposes the sufferer in his vulnerability covers him with a sense of shameful resourcelessness. Thus the parents of the retarded and the handicapped and the accident victim need help in identifying those resources still theirs and in learning how to draw on them.

The chapter on the Dax case so emphasized the patient's loss that it failed to underscore the importance of taking an inventory of what remains. This continuity of resources, however, does not soften the experience of break in identity or lessen the necessity of acquiring a new identity. The recovery of resources does not usually let one merely reassert one's old self intact as though nothing had intervened. Parents, for example, may need a reordered sense of themselves to recognize a now-valuable resource which they had previously relegated to the basement or the attic of their lives. Traits of character hardly required before the arrival of the retarded now loom large in helping the parents cope. And their gratifications also change. Accomplishments hardly noticed in the ordinary child now deserve a prize. One may still miss the allegro passages in rearing a child but the largo passages begin to acquire some subtlety for the retrained ear.

The term "transition" evokes the metaphor of a journey; and no pilgrim manages a difficult journey without some virtues that assist the passage. Loyalty heads the list of those virtues which a fully realized bonding requires: a double loyalty, to both the being and the well-being of the child. Parental loyalty, as noted later in this chapter, requires both. Neither loyalty is complete without the other. Both loyalties also require their own differing forms of the virtue of courage. Full pursuit of the child's well-being requires that "active" courage which Thomas Aquinas associated with "attack," the courage to overcome daunting obstacles which the parents of the retarded or the otherwise handicapped face in abundance. But loyal acceptance of the child's being, his existence as he is, requires that "passive" courage which Thomas associated with "endurance," the capacity to perdure in the midst of obstacles only some of which will yield to attack.

Bonding parents also require the virtue of justice, inasmuch as loyalty turns destructive without the constraint of justice. Left to itself, love responds without stint to the needs of another, but love diminishes into a sentiment less than just and, ultimately, less than loving if it fails to satisfy the legitimate claims of third parties. Specifically, love directed to the boundless needs of the retarded can sacrifice yet other members of the family. Justice requires some measure of equality in family life. However, equal treatment does not mean identical treatment. Justice defined as identical treatment blocks love's need to respond to specific needs. It foolishly misses the target when the differences between children in a family are great. Equal treatment in a family ought more appropriately to mean making an equal contribution to the good in the life of each member. This ideal lets the content of that contribution take different forms depending upon differing needs. It would remind sharply the retarded's parents of their equal but differing responsibilities to each of their children. Undoubtedly the sheer magnitude of the retarded's needs makes it difficult to accommodate tidily to the claims of justice in the distribution of love, but the claim of justice reminds parents that even as love does its best, it must also apportion at its best.

Other virtues must come into play, including a wisdom that distinguishes the important from the unimportant and the doable from the impossible. But whatever the virtues required along the way, bonding takes hold in the parents when the event they originally perceived as blank and intractable fate now seizes them as destiny, in which they imperfectly but humanly find their identity and calling.

Attachment. Healthy attachment presupposes a number of prenatal and immediate postnatal activities that support bonding. The mother, clearly, and the father in some instances also, can engage in: (a) prior to pregnancy, at least some touching of babies (even if only by babysitting); (b) during pregnancy, feeling the fetus kick (the perception of the fetus as a separate individual sometimes converts unwanted to more acceptable or wanted pregnancies); (c) witnessing birth (studies suggest that those who witness birth are more likely to bond to the child than those who do not); (d) immediate cuddling after birth (parents deprived of access to the baby during the so-called sensitive period, are inclined to be less attached; the baby "belongs," as it were, to someone else); (e) setting up a favorable institutional setting (homelike, if not at home, with professional staff assisting, rather than displacing, the mother); (f) reciprocally interacting (touch, eye-to-eye contact—the child can see at birth), talking (the neonate prefers the high-pitched female voice), entraining (a type of dance movement in the course of conversation between mother and child), smelling (by the fifth day a baby can tell its mother's breast pad), sensing (heat, and heartbeat)—to say nothing of absorbing the bacterial nasal flora and antibodies imparted with the mother's milk.[17]

We can interpret the proposal that final attachment to the retarded child resembles induction into the sacred in traditional societies either sentimentally or realistically. Sentimental testimony abounds. One parent professes, "I believe a brain-injured child is a gift from God. This child is a precious gift to the family."[18] Another parent avers, "The child we have is like an angel. Treat him well, he will put in a good word for us with God."[19] Medieval people sometimes referred to the retarded as "infants of the good God"[20]—and allowed them special freedom to roam. The fool, we know, enjoyed a measure of liberty in the royal court denied to others. This special elevation of the retarded reflects itself in the very word sometimes used to designate them: cretin. Although the word has now fallen into disuse or smacks of the pejorative, some suggest that it derives from the word "Christian." At one time, the retarded alone seemed to deserve the adjective "Christian" so often loosely (and wrongly) used to suggest innocence. Owing to their simplicity of mind, the retarded alone seemed incorruptible.

Such views verge on the sentimental. The phrase "gift of God" sometimes functions less as a theological assertion than as a claim about some inevitably good consequence that follows from the birth of a retarded child. It claims too much for the retarded's tonic impact on its family and society. It smacks too much, albeit poignantly, of the fervent rhetoric that one sometimes hears from AA and other support groups that need missionary zeal in order to sustain courage. Gifts from God —some retarded children surely may seem, but they are not inevitably so received or perceived. Taking responsibility for the retarded may deepen lives in some families. But suffering does not always ennoble. Heavy responsibilities can crush as well as strengthen their bearers.

Yet, parents and children do bond, and sometimes so deeply that the bonding powerfully transforms life. Another parent resorts to religious language: "A child like this is a sacrament." The parent thereby concedes that caring for an abnormal child makes one feel "outcast, doomed somehow not to be normal oneself," but acknowledges, at the same time, "an entirely different covenant with existence."[21] In another instance, the father of an autistic child rages against his lot and yet finally concedes: "Consciousness is like a free gift arising out of a bond that is tragic and good. But for him, I guess, and for us, the bond is what comes first."[22]

Words such as "tragic," "doomed," "outcast" still appear in the testimony, however. But the harshness of the experience no longer overwhelms. Parents and child have attached. Featherstone wryly acknowledges a negative sign of this bonding. "At the minimum and wintry level, acceptance may begin to bring the recognition that the child's hardship no longer represents the only obstacle to happiness."[23] Still, bonding can eventually bring rewards: the brother of a mildly retarded busboy reports taking stock of his deficient sibling. A stranger innocently asks him the rather conventional question—What does your brother do for a living? The young man, for the first time, does not answer preemptively by explaining that his brother, because retarded, works only as a menial in a restaurant. "Suddenly it struck me for the first time in the twenty-eight years of our lives together that mental slowness is not the sum of [my brother's] existence. He is a man who is married, holds down a job, pays taxes." So he returns to the question and simply tells the stranger, "He's in the restaurant business!"[24]

The literature on the retarded child usually closes with a discussion of "acceptance." However, acceptance does not describe the bonded parent without qualification. Attachment, at its deepest level, sets up a tension between acceptance of the child as it is and a quest for interventions that will improve his lot. Any human being bonded to the being and well-being of another does what he can and enlists the aid of others to serve its good. Simple acceptance alone hardly describes the parents' relationship to their child as they attempt what they can to foster their child's excellence and well-being. To that end, of course, they seek the services of the doctor and, eventually, the teacher—to stretch the child's capacities and to help it live up to them.

However, a compulsion to act can turn demonic, hammering the child with help that rejects the child as it is. It may also betray a profound self-rejection. The parent feels guilty about having produced a child with defects and attempts to atone by becoming a superparent. Sooner or later, the parent must reckon with and accept the child's limits. Otherwise, the effort to serve the child's excellence and well-being deteriorates into a battering and self-battering masked beneath the fair face of love.

Attachment needs both activism and acceptance. Religiously put: attachment becomes too quietistic if it slackens into mere acceptance of the child as it is. Love must will the well-being and not merely the being of the other. But, even worse, attachment lapses into a gnostic revulsion against the world if in the name of well-being it recoils from the child in its deprived state of being. One observer perceived the right balance between acceptance and intervention when he observed, "I admire the purpose and ingenuity with which parents and children forge a good life out of imperfect materials."[25] Attachment includes efforts at transformation, yes; but not as though all value rests in the transformation, as though the transformation must surpass the imperfect materials themselves for anything good to come of the life.

Valuing. We misunderstand valuing the retarded child if we place value wholly in the marketplace. By "marketplace" I mean a setting in which we treat the retarded child as a discrete item in the world, to be compared and weighed against other discrete items. In this setting, one asks what correlations appear between natural ability and perceived worth and then one tests out that worth by deciding on how many social resources (public and familiar) one will spend to support and enhance the retarded. What price, in effect, can the retarded command within the public and domestic economy? This question, so formulated, begs for an answer in the coin of utility.

This approach misses the issue in valuing not so much because it judges cruelly and ruthlessly (though it often does) but because it misses the even more cruel question which the retarded themselves pose. The retarded do not chiefly pose the question "What is the relative worth, or lack of it, of a child with my particular disabilities?" They ask, rather "What worth has a world that includes me in it?" Parents also face the latter, more encompassing, metaphysical question. This child, my child, not the child I hoped for, named, and registered for college in fancy, depresses for me utterly the world's worth. Herein lies the deep quarrel with God, the terrible envy and resentment of friends. Parents face not the problem of relative good in a marketplace of goods and preferences, but the problem of evil. The arrival of the deprived child raises the question of the worth of the world and the worthwhileness of life. The question deepens and darkens beyond the perceived worth of the child relative to other goods, to the worth of anything whatsoever. Nothing seems worth a candle. Do the powers that matter in life impoverish and crush, or do they bless?

Parents see the problem at this more metaphysical level because they suffer at this level. And, at least some of them, it would appear, have sought to respond at this level when they have confessed themselves to feel outcast and doomed and yet have reckoned with the child as establishing their "covenant with existence." Bonding to a child who renders questionable the value of existence reestablishes one's covenant with existence. Neither policy-makers nor professionals should deal with that testimony lightly.[26]

This covenant with existence demands devotion beyond the ordinary measure. Featherstone likens the plight of parents to the person who happens upon a drowning man. As the only person there, she can jump in and try to save him, or she can agonize on shore. "In the first case I am a hero; in the second, a coward. There is no way I can remain what I was before—an ordinary person."[27] But heroism alone does not sustain the covenant; the child also sustains the parents. That sustenance may be difficult to acknowledge without sounding as though one justifies the retardation. Yet some parents have acknowledged the deepening of their lives; they find themselves in retrospect a little kinder, a little gentler, a little more sensitive to the difficulties others face than they might otherwise have been.[28]

Because this is the case, valuing the retarded does not arbitrarily place a pricetag on an imperfect product that someone has manufactured. Valuing persons differs from inventing, fabricating, and marketing things. It discovers and honors what is already there; it does not merely impute; and therefore, reciprocally, this valuing, which opens to the value of the other, also imparts strength to those who do the valuing.

Values are not ideal demands alone; they also affirm and define strength and power. The Latin root for value—*valere*—from which we also derive valor and valid and convalescent—implies this affirmation. The convalescent whom illness has assaulted begins to grow again in strength. The valorous man or woman faces adversity strongly, stoutly, bravely, vigorously, and powerfully. The brave person exudes power in the face of odds.

Similarly, when we refer to values—to the value of the family, work, love, birth, and the retarded child—we talk, not about frothy matters that we imagine or invent, but about people, institutions, ideals, and demands that bear down upon us. They validate themselves, as it were, as stout, strong, vigorous, and powerful, prevailing upon us as worthy of response in our freedom. Values elicit commitments from which, in turn, strength and power derive.

AN EPILOGUE ON POLICIES
AND QUANDARIES

This essay has tried to put the problem of valuing the retarded in a relational setting. It has looked to the relationship between parents and child for its clue to moral claims and obligations. It has attended specifically to the process of bonding, as it honors and values another and as it generates loyalty and trust between those bonded. The path to bonding does not usually run smooth. Parents undergo an ordeal that beggars description except in the language reserved for induction into the sacred. The testimony of parents reminds one of the language that one associates with the relational thinkers. Kierkegaard spoke of fear and trembling in the God-relationship;[29] Heidegger reckoned with dread in the relationship to death;[30] Buber recognized that the "I" and the "Thou" remain strange to one another in the very midst of I-Thou address.[31] Relationship to the retarded at the deepest level requires a transformation that upsets, winnows, confuses, and turns around the self.

The use of this religious language also implies that the process of bonding affects more than psychological being; it affects us ontologically and morally; bonding gives a clue to the being and well-being of others, to one's obligation to them, and to one's own being and value in so honoring the tie.

This general approach departs from the prevailing tendency among moralists to resort exclusively to the notion of abstract rights and duties in dealing with the moral warrants for care of the retarded. Ethicists usually begin with natural capacities (such as intelligence) abstracted from the historical accidents of family, religion, education, and the like, and seek to determine what duties we owe to all human beings who possess and show these capacities. This approach has led, across the last century and a half, to establishing huge facilities designed to care for people who, by virtue of natural misfortune or historical accident, suffer abuse or neglect at the hands of their fellows or who need care of a kind which neither they nor their families nor their friends can offer. The support for these institutions—hospitals, mental hospitals, nursing homes, and workshops—comes largely from strangers (through taxation or philanthropic giving); further, they are manned by strangers, whose job it is to give help to strangers (to all persons whatsoever, irrespective of ties).

The approach taken in this essay differs (but only partly) from this prevailing view of rights and duties and its institutional results. The generation of a set of rights and duties to the retarded by abstractly considering natural abilities leads to moral minimalism and to a minimal discharge of those duties in huge institutions. Duties based on rights tend to diminish to whatever a socially undefined person can enforce against anybody. We write off additional obligations that grow from bonding as merely optional and preferential. These optional obligations enter into discussion of what the society owes creatures whose being and worth disclose themselves chiefly in the context of ties. The disquieting results of this minimalism are all about us in a rootless and libertarian post-Enlightenment society. We reduced our direct obligations toward the marginal and the deviant, and discharge those few obligations we acknowledge through the device of segregative institutions and isolative services. The retarded's right to these services and the shape we have given them result from a bondless consideration of natural abilities and worth. Meanwhile, the very scale and structure of the institutions themselves have made it more difficult to bond within their walls.

A more relational approach does not, however, argue for the dismantling of large-scale institutions. Criticism ought not obscure either the philanthropic impulse that often prompted their founding or the conscientious efforts of many of their managers and staff to calibrate their limited resources to real needs. Moreover, some versions of mainstreaming today set the needy free from segregated institutions only to abandon them to the *de facto* segregation of third-rate hotels or the streets and tunnels of a city. Care deteriorates from little to nothing.

At the policy level, a respect for the importance of bonding should encourage the reform rather than the dissolution of total institutions. It should highlight those various factors that foster and nurture small-scale community even in large institutional settings—architectural design, the layout of interior space, equipment, public and private rooms, and the strategic use of professional teams and volunteer groups. Further, a respect for bonding should encourage the society to provide some mildly or moderately retarded persons with more small-scale communities (surrogate families) as an alternative residential choice to either the large-scale institution or the family home. Such facilities would also lessen the trauma institutional residents face when the society mainstreams them (only too often a euphemism for drifting and crashing amongst the shoals and reefs of big-city life). Finally, it should also encourage more adequate public support to families to ease the burden of family care—more adequate training programs, respite houses that provide families with periodic relief from total care, and the mobilization of religious and other volunteer groups to supplement the nuclear family with some of those resources previously available only through the extended family.

Such strategic assistance to families helps at two points. It encourages more families to keep their children at home rather than commit them to institutions. It also lessens the traumas both the retarded and their families face if and as the society mainstreams more of the mildly or moderately retarded and thrusts them back into their homes. The family that receives back a deinstitutionalized child after having lived on its own needs help as it reabsorbs the child into the family.

Even though it might improve social policies and render less harsh the choices parents must make, a more relational approach will not solve all quandaries parents face: whether to institutionalize a child; what goods will best serve the well-being of a child; what balance to strike between the claims of the retarded child and those of other siblings, work, and marriage. Indeed, bonding often intensifies rather than solves problems in casuistry. The bonded agent must reckon with conflicting loyalties, not just competing preferences, when reaching a decision. He cannot, moreover, blunt the moral ache of the decision by resort to the marketplace device of calculating tradeoffs or balancing goods over evils. He must honor the tragic, or, as religious people may prefer, the divine comedic element in a moral decision. A decision to institutionalize does not merely add a debit to a balance. One persists in wishing otherwise, even when one chooses one's course. The brokenness, the incompleteness, the tragedy, the poignancy of a decision moves with us into the future—unless an ultimate perspective with more depth than a balance sheet lets us see things whole.

Finally, a relational approach cannot seriously claim to derive notions of worth wholly from the faulty testimony of those who bond to one another. If worth depends upon a human tie alone, the retarded child is wholly hostage to the erratic valuations of parents and caregivers, good, bad or indifferent. That is why Enlightenment moralists tried to establish a notion of worth irrespective of ties. Their minimalism sought to prevent worse fates. The external and internal obstacles to bonding and the awesome process of detachment, transition, and attachment must give one pause about placing authority for making ultimate judgments of worth in the hands of parents and others who face, many times unsuccessfully, that difficult ordeal. The battered child silences foolish sentimentality about the success rate of bonding. If value and the perception of value derive entirely from a relationship, then the powerless one within the relationship becomes wholly hostage to it. Parents cannot claim to be the sole or final arbiters of the value of their children. Frail and facing a process strewn with obstacles, parents do not always bond well or wisely. This consideration and caution partly led the theological tradition, when speaking relationally, to posit a God-relationship as encompassing, authorizing, judging, and forgiving all others. To testify, however, to that relationship with bonded conviction, one must suffer an induction into the sacred—of which the ordeals I have described in this essay offer a petty parable and sign.

THE RETARDED
INSTITUTIONALIZED

A PARTICIPANT AT A conference on mental retardation heard me confess my lack of contact with the retarded in institutions and deftly called my hand. She invited me to attend a three-day session, called Inside Out, at the Caswell Center for the Retarded in Kinston, North Carolina. Only her smile revealed what both of us knew. She had neatly bagged me. I agreed to come if I could.

I doubted, however, that the experience would satisfy the canons of investigative journalism or anthropological field research. Several days in a state facility—days carefully planned for visitors, largely college students—would probably be inside-out, but also best-foot-forward. A controlled experience at best. The sheer numbers of visitors would partially displace the atmosphere of the facility.

Still, I went ahead with the visit, arriving in Kinston at 3:30 P.M. with orientation to begin at 4:00. Earl Williams, a black in his thirties, soft-spoken, cultured, in charge of recruiting volunteers for the Center, met me. He works with churches and other groups. Ideal for the job, a native of the area, he married a school sweetheart who teaches English at the local high school. Williams worked as a resident advocate for eight months before switching to his current job. He originally planned to move to the North, but the cost of living chilled that plan. On the side, he is finishing a seminary degree with plans for the Baptist ministry. Life is on an upward curve for Earl Williams.

We toured the grounds in his car before he deposited me for the sessions. The large campus offered the older buildings first, built on a family-cottage scale. They were appropriate for what he called a "paternalistic model" of care. Each unit had in earlier days a resident mother and father. But later "we started to warehouse them" in the bigger and newer facilities. Still farther along, he pointed out the most recent buildings, where Caswell Center keeps the severely and profoundly retarded who are also afflicted with various physical handicaps. They were cared for on a more "medical model." I did not look forward to a visit to that unit.

My hostess greeted me warmly at the registration desk, conveying a touch of surprise that I had actually shown up but glad that I had. Immediately, she took me to a location where I was to leave my luggage under lock and key. "We take luggage away from our visitors immediately and ask them to park their cars in a fenced-off compound in order to let them experience what it's like to enter into a total institution. Residents lose control over their own property." "I don't tell the student visitors that," she confided. "We want them to discover for themselves that they have been dispossessed."

My colleagues in this experience? Chiefly special education students at East Carolina University and other institutions in the state; about 45 all told.

The director of Caswell Center, at that time, Rick Zaharia, gave the opening talk. He promptly mentioned Erving Goffman's *Total Institutions*, "the most important book you can read about an institution like this: what it means to eat, sleep, live, work in a single inclusive campus facility which encloses all its residents and distinguishes, first and foremost, the inside from the outside—the world out there." Zaharia was making a deliberate effort to create a more open institution. "Inside Outside" was part of that attempt. Not that Zaharia had any illusions: "You will see the warts on our nose, the downside of life, but also, perhaps, a few exhilarating moments. I urge you to sneak off from the group and its planned sessions from time to time to see what you please for yourself. No doors are locked during the day, only after dark. When I see you at the end of your stay, I hope that you will have some tough questions. They pay me a lot to take the heat." Our leaders, responsible for a battalion of college students, were not enthusiastic about the invitation to improvise on the schedule.

The first evening we would take the easy way into the water, at the shallow and warm end of the pool. We received conventional information about mental retardation, the usual distinctions between the mildly retarded who are educable, the moderately retarded who can function in "sheltered workshops," and the severely and profoundly retarded who compose the vast majority of residents in a facility like this. Programs for deinstitutionalization have mainstreamed most of the mildly and moderately retarded into group homes, their original family settings, or the culture at large. A gentle movie about group homes, "A Family of Friends," followed Zaharia's lecture. The state of North Carolina maintains 85 to 100 group homes.

A note about supper, cafeteria style. If I didn't know I was in a total institution, I knew it then. Early (5:00 P.M.) suppers in hospitals and other facilities, whatever else they accomplish, serve the convenience of staff. They put the day to bed early and let the staff go home. We ate in the staff refectory but received common fare. The food built up in my stomach a solid column of starch. Bottom layer, the bun of a sloppy joe; just to the north of that a substantial portion of high-density beans; then, canned corn, topped off by a glaze layer-cake for dessert. My student colleagues tackled the food without scruple. In fact, some of them found a supply of potato chips to provide well-nigh total coverage of the staple carbohydrates. These students were a switch from the lean suburban types I am accustomed to seeing on college campuses. On the strength of supper, I expected the retarded who are able to feed themselves to be well-larded.

Mrs. Lacewell, a black, gave the most successful talk of the evening, a slide presentation called "My Special Friends." It featured mildly retarded residents, increasingly an anachronism in the institution now that mainstreaming policies prevail. Residents are aware of the difference. They refer to themselves as high-grade and low-grade. Al was in a low-grade facility, but he always dressed up and wore a tie. Even though nonverbal, he was saying, in effect, that he wasn't low-grade.

Miscellaneous advice from our leaders: You must not breach confidentiality by betraying the identity of a resident to the outside world or by sharing information about an already identified person. You must sign a confidentiality agreement and can be sued if you violate it. (All names of residents and, with one exception, of residence halls have been changed in this report.) You can shake hands with residents, but if a resident hugs you or drapes himself or herself on you, don't permit it. They have to learn appropriate behavior. It's their best protection if they venture into the outside world. If they hug strangers outside, they will get into trouble.

Only 10 percent of the residents are mildly or moderately retarded (high-functioning). Most are severely or profoundly retarded. Almost 900 of the 1000 residents are adult. We will see lots of physical disability among the low-functioning. They will look alike to us, but eventually we will be able to distinguish them.

Time to go to our sleeping quarters—in my case, the residence hall for severely and profoundly retarded men. I talked briefly with the night staff before going to bed. Three blacks and a white. The white man chattily assumed the role as spokesman to this white visitor from the outside world. One sees such preemptive behavior in New York City all the time. On a subway platform a white man will choose to ask his questions of another white man in preference to blacks nearer by, as though only whites had a public identity or competence. All staff members conceded, however, that one of the blacks was most adept with the residents. He alone had a way with them, could get them to do what he wanted. The official floor leader, a black woman, registered (but without whining) a complaint I was to hear several times over: staff members had to write up endless reports on each of the patients. As far as she could see, it consumed too much time without much point. I got to bed around midnight. Residents were up and about at 5:00 in the morning. Staff members and cleaning crews seemed to talk all night. I assume that residents get used to it. Most of them sleep with the doors open to the hallway.

I left for breakfast the next morning in the rain with two colleagues. Squads of residents were in the hallway. I shook hands with the person nearby who offered his hand; but as I passed I realized that a number of other residents offered their hands, and I, in the momentum of walking out with my colleagues, a little late for breakfast, shook hands only with the one, as though he were deputy for the rest. I regretted that incident as much as any in the course of my visit. I should have stayed and shook hands with them all.

After breakfast we broke up into groups of six or seven and started on our respective tours of the facilities. We stopped first at a "low-functioning" unit—one of the large buildings where, as my first contact, Earl Williams, had said, Caswell had formerly "warehoused" patients. Our guide now explained that they don't use the terms low-grade and high-grade anymore, it's low-functioning and high-functioning. Here one found women whose chronological ages ran from 13 to 44 years but who were sometimes only 8 months or even less in mental age. The residence hall happened at this hour to be empty. The residents were in training classes in another building. "We try to train them, though they're not toilet trained. We teach them to grasp objects. Caswell Center holds an annual conference on each resident where we determine their needs and training regimen."

To qualify for higher levels of funding under Medicaid, state governments have converted former custodial bins into intermediate care facilities that mandate training for each resident. Residents now spend six hours a day in an active training program. But the leader admitted that institutions have gradually broadened the meaning of compliance with this regulation. Residents, both those whose experience at the facility preceded the training program and those who came out of families where they had no training whatsoever, felt badgered by so much training. Even quiet time is now interpreted as part of the training. What qualified quiet time as training? The fact that it is scheduled.

Even those who can't move get training. For them, it may mean simply moving parts of their bodies. Many residents are nonverbal, therefore staff members communicate with them by pointing to pictures pasted on a board. One picture shows a toilet, the others a bed, a TV set, a wash-basin, a dining table, or the outdoors.

Only one resident in the "low-functioning" unit was on the floor —literally. A young woman of 20 or so kept rocking herself on a chair, then crouched ducklike, moving impatiently to and fro. Tiring of that, she lay down on the floor, banging her head on the ground and making flatulent noises with her mouth. I wondered why she didn't wear a helmet for protection, like several helmeted residents I had seen in my sleeping facility. One of our leaders had explained to me earlier that the helmeted residents, more than likely, were not head-bangers but epileptics who had up to thirty fits a day. Thirty meant thirty falls to the ground in which they were likely to damage themselves—above and beyond the damage already wrought by the electrical storm in their heads. (A later visit to the Kennedy Institute for Handicapped Children at Johns Hopkins University raised doubts as to whether a fit, apart from the fall, injures an epileptic. A physician there said it is a debated point.)

The "low-functioning" unit had recently been remodeled from a warehouse facility, consisting of a large dormitory room with from forty to sixty beds, into an intermediate care facility. It was now divided into six separate bedrooms with four residents to a bedroom. Residents had individual beds and a two-drawer half-width chest about the size of a bedtable. But these residents had no more sense of their own property and clothes than does a four-month-old baby. They eat in the facility. To preserve privacy, staff members give them a shower and dry them off one at a time. A house staff member mentioned going on a trip with a somewhat higher-functioning resident. When she proceeded to towel the young woman after the shower, the resident quickly twirled her body around. Obviously, residents were trained to twirl and speed up the routine as other residents waited in line for their showers.

Low-functioning residents in a training center spend their time screwing nuts into a board, sorting coins, or performing other elementary tasks. This so-called occupational therapy for low-functioning people doesn't actually train them for a job, but offers quite primitive but important physical training. For example, they may learn to control their tongues (to limit slobbering) or to regulate some muscle movement. Staff members also saw value in their going to a different building for school; it kept them from spending the whole of their lives in one building. Everyone reported on the stark contrast between buildings with and buildings without intermediate care facility funding.

Many of the teachers, trainers, and "recreators" at Caswell Center are black people. I appreciate now John Jacobs's remark (as successor to Vernon Jordan of the Urban League) that the Reagan federal budget cuts not only drastically reduced services to poor blacks but also eliminated many jobs for educated blacks. Jacobs observed that 50 percent of educated blacks work for the government—federal, state, or local. Reagan's budget cuts affected the black community irrespective of economic and social class.

We visited yet another residential facility in which the residents were off to a training center. This time, a building for adolescent boys. The matron proudly cited the level of group discipline they had achieved. Except for one boy whose mother visits once a month, the rest see a relative about once a year. Each bed was made and some kind of stuffed animal decorated the bed. In yet another residence, the staff, in an effort to allow the residents "age-appropriate" behavior, have permitted nude pin-ups to replace stuffed bears.

I had a morning appointment with Zaharia on the background of the institution. In 1964, Caswell Center had 2,053 clients and 1,600 staff members; in 1976, 1,450 clients and 1,000 staff members; in 1982, 1,069 clients and 1,700 staff members. In 1982 there were five back-up personnel—grounds crew, dining hall workers, etc.—for every "hands-on" professional. Federal funding made possible the more favorable ratio of client population to staff size at Caswell. The campus had increased the number of hands-on caregivers to residents from 1:60 to 1:6. Intermediate care facility funding had increased from 90 federally funded beds in 1976 to 600 such beds in 1982. The state of North Carolina funded beds at the level of $55 a day but the federal government at $75 a day (1982). The $20-a-bed extra through ICF funding paid for the good things that Caswell was able to do beyond the warehousing of inmates. Staff members expected Reagan's cutbacks to change this, but by 1990, Caswell still had over 1,700 staff members, serving but 847 clients with ICF funding for 743 beds. The federal government thus covers $45 million of the $54 million annual budget at the Center.

"What is the lead problem that you face at Caswell, the problem least amenable to solution?" I asked. "Rural North Carolina has trouble getting physicians. We should have six physicians on our staff but the best we have done is four physicians and, of course, often they are foreign-born, they cannot speak English, and when they learn it they leave. We have contracted with the East Carolina University Medical School for pediatric services ($25,000) and pay out $50,000 in fees for specialists. We are able to get free services from the Dorothea Dix psychiatric facility in Raleigh. We hope that the new medical school at East Carolina University, which emphasizes the training of family practitioners and gives preference to local applicants for medical school, will eventually ease the problem of medical staffing."

Dental care. "We have a total staff of two-persons-plus. That gives us a ratio of 1 dentist to 500 patients, not the optimal 1 to 200. Local dentists and physicians provide services." (In 1990, medical and dental support remained at approximately the same levels.)

While recognizing that his comment was mildly self-serving, Zaharia observed that it was better not to have a physician as head of the Caswell Center because it would tend to medicalize the facility. He also felt it important for the person to have some professional education and experience in running an organization of this size. Zaharia had received his master's degree in educational psychology with a later dissertation in special administration at the Peabody Institute in Nashville. Thereafter he made his way up through the ranks in institutions like the Caswell Center.

The chaplain, Roy Cyr, who had a B.D. from Duke and a master's degree in special education and had moved into the chaplaincy out of a staff job in special education at the Center, saw his primary duty as pastoral care for residents. (I found him in this respect a refreshing change from some chaplains I have known in universities who grow weary of students and eventually redefine their jobs as primarily service to faculty members of their own age.) Cyr holds services on Sundays and a short "worship experience" in halls for those who can't come for service to the large and visually blank sanctuary. Chaplain Cyr attempts to establish links between residents and church members in the Kinston community and hopes to organize church people for some services at Caswell Center. He views work with the family as important, since families, as well as the retarded, suffer when a son or daughter, brother or sister, leaves home for the institution. Cyr has organized some of the higher-functioning residents to visit sick residents or to attend local churches.

Back to the tour. We visited a prevocational center where high-functioning residents receive training and learn to work with small hand tools. Since their attention span is limited, they work for one to three hours each day. The DuPont Company contracts for the work they do, which is bona fide, not busy work. They get paid on a prorated basis, scaled down to their level of productivity compared with normal workers.

Our last stop was Omega, the building that housed the profoundly retarded and multiply handicapped. Earl Williams had pointed it out to me on our opening tour of the campus. The last letter of the Greek alphabet seemed a fitting symbol. Omega stood at the end of the line, the segregated institution within the segregated institution, where the distorted, the disfigured, and the twisted sit in tailor-made contraptions, ingenious wheelchair mechanisms, or manage an occasional "spider," an adult-child's walker. The bathrooms in Omega had specially designed tubs that must have cost many thousands of dollars. One tub had a huge foam ring about it to keep spastics from hurting themselves. All tubs had expensive devices to help staff lift patients in and out and to keep the patients from slipping and falling. I asked whether bathing was the high point of the day as it was for some babies, but staff told me that some residents resist bathing. It must be a slippery, eelish business. Most residents here cannot feed themselves, but a special "AC feeder" assists people with cerebral palsy: the patient-resident leans over and gets food off a mechanized spoon-scoop. I felt somewhat relieved as we left Omega, but, my speculation about symbols to the contrary, I had not yet seen the worst: the profoundly retarded and multiply handicapped children were located in the Alpha building.

Because of my background in religious studies, the leaders of the conference had arranged for me to meet Ben Ranseur, the director of religious services. On the way over, I watched residents make their way along the long canopied sidewalks between buildings. The lame, the halt, and the blind would help one another, sometimes making use of an iron hand railing that ran the length of the walk. The scraping noise of steel on the pavement announced the slow progress along the walk of a man whose leg tendons were so drawn up that he could not place his feet flat on the ground. He used the hand rail as he moved forward, his feet peddling, as it were, in slow motion, rather than walking. Each leg described a kind of ellipse of its own, but since his feet could neither lie flat nor lift off the ground, he had to drag himself forward on his toes. Someone had shod the front of his shoes, both top and bottom, with steel to make possible his heroic passage.

Ranseur's education in music and his bluff, outgoing, energetic manner, effective in rough-and-tumble with the higher functioning residents, probably got him the job. The choir sings in community churches. One appearance there, he said, "can wipe away years of inappropriate attitudes toward MR's." I had visions of Bertolt Brecht's Promenade of the Cripples in the Berliner Ensemble production of the *Threepenny Opera* in East Berlin. Ranseur, like Cyr, emphasized that he works with residents more than with staff or the outside community. My question to him: "In addition to fulfilling your pastoral duties, do you sometimes see yourself as fulfilling an advisory, critical, sometimes adversarial role at the institution?" "Yes," he said. "For example, all surgery for residents gets done at Dorothea Dix in Raleigh, North Carolina, free of charge. Until recently, Dorothea Dix Hospital had the practice of calling up the Center only the night before an operation to warn the resident and relevant staff member of the procedure. We had no time to prepare the resident for the experience." Apparently Dorothea Dix used the Caswell Center as a filler for unexpected breaks in the schedule. So Ranseur took up the issue with the social worker at Dorothea Dix and eventually got the policies changed. It was agreed that Caswell Center would receive five days' notice of scheduled surgery or, if on shorter notice, the call would come as an invitation rather than a command.

I had noticed, in passing, a sign on the Omega facility that advised staff members to report broken bones not only to the director of the facility but also to the advocate's office maintained by the central administration. This rule may be a self-protective measure, but, at the same time, it suggests an effort to build some critical review of services into the system.

An interview with Hampton Carmine, in charge of program observation, covered some of the earlier history of the institution, but also helped me get hold of a central issue.

Caswell maintained centralized control over all professional services. It had 1,800 to 2,000 residents and only 300 residents were in training programs. Caswell then broke up into smaller managerial units, placing more professionals on staff and putting them closer to the residents as the institution decentralized into divisions distinguished by age and level of functioning.

Judy Kurzer, now working at the Western Carolina Center for the Retarded, pushed for major changes at Caswell. (Perhaps she never got the big job because she was too controversial?) Kurzer hired directors, who, like herself, had a background in social work, to head each of the eight divisions. Caswell owes the major reforms to her and, of course, to later federal financing.

A looming moral problem. "I have 55 residents in my charge, only 15 of whom will be significantly altered by what I do. The principle of fairness, however forbids a policy of helping only the 15. Everyone should get something. Therefore my colleagues and I try to educate everybody. To enforce and support that effort, we insist on documentation for every resident. We have volumes on everybody. As interventionists rather than custodians, we must have a plan for progress and report on that progress. Previously, not even staff members could see the record, such as it was, on each patient. Now records are decentralized and accessible to all relevant parties. These policies reflect an institution more therapeutic than custodial in orientation."

But now to the problem. "When you must show the client's progress, you tend to emphasize what you can measure; and you can measure the performance of tasks, such as putting bolts in holes, more readily than social attitudes and interactions. This facility, like most other conscientious facilities today, aims at and measures performance. It is more difficult to measure emotional needs and progress in attaining emotional stability and rapport. The system doesn't make it easy to direct time and resources to more elusive social goals. Do you measure units of smiling to get at happiness? It would sound as though we were teaching smiling.

"Further, training the higher functioning to perform tasks can bore not just the staff but also the residents. Boredom adversely affects the development of social skills. Caswell, after all, is already a massively routinized institution. We live by the clock. The hours of repeated activity needed to make progress in the performance of a task increases the amount of routine in their lives. And routine kills talk! If you are fed at the same time every day you don't have to say that you're hungry. [I thought of the links between routine and taciturnity in marriage.]"

The relentless routine of institutional life plus the constant training in motor skills plunges residents still further into the nonverbal. Both residents and staff become less creative. Training oriented to perform- ance also fails to address the more primitive social needs of residents at still lower levels of functioning. Hectoring at the hands of a trainer is often less relevant to their condition than simple touching and cra- dling.

In a talk later that day, Gerry Lyle, administrator for the in-services network in the state, noted the difference that President Kennedy made in the care of the retarded in this country. Before Kennedy, the govern- ment spent only 3 to 20 dollars a day on their care. Increasingly, now, the state is making an effort to relocate the retarded, by transferring the more capable out of a cathedral institution like Caswell and into a home or group setting. Twenty percent of the people at Caswell would not be admitted there today because of changed criteria for admission. While the policy of deinstitutionalizing has removed from total institu- tions some people who should not be there, it has often thrown on their own resources or into overloaded institutions, such as the nuclear family, persons who either should have remained in total institutions or who need more intermediate assistance than our society has yet been willing to supply them. Community services need to expand to support deinstitutionalization.[1]

My special assignment for an extended visit turned out to be Alpha House, where the multiply handicapped and profoundly retarded chil- dren reside. Staff members find it most difficult to handle those cases of children born normal who have suffered severe brain damage from a car accident or high fever. One child smashed her head in a car accident at two years of age. Her parents brought her to the Center at five years of age; she then weighed 16 pounds. Now, at age ten, she weighs 35 pounds. Her foster grandparent at the facility had her spread-eagled out on a huge, colored beach ball about three and a half feet in circum- ference. (I assumed the intent was recreational, and probably in part it was; later, at the Kennedy Institute for the Handicapped at Johns Hopkins, I learned that the staff there uses such balls to teach cerebral palsy victims—and others—muscular equilibrium. The huge beach ball gives more distributed support than arm-holding, and yet allows, as staff moves it, shifts in the center of gravity to which the body must adjust. Those who have little sense of equilibrium and muscular control do not get the human reassurance from being held that others do. Hold- ing with just two hands is too pinpointed. Everything else splays, the child goes floppy and out of control. The emotional consequences of this for family intimacy must be enormous.) Some hydrocephalics couldn't hold up their heads, others lay on pallets where their foster grandparents rubbed them. Still others wore helmets. The service contraptions ran the gamut I had already seen in Omega House.

Foster grandparents are older people of modest means living in the area who spend four hours a day at the facility. They get paid on an hourly basis and receive one meal a day. Assigned to spend two hours with one child and then two hours with the second, they hold, caress, engage in simple play, and feed each child one of their three meals for the day, thus reducing the burden of feeding for full-time staff. Across a four-hour stint, a grandparent feeds one of her children breakfast, the other, lunch. Not that eating means what it ordinarily does for normal children of their age. All children there eat soft foods only. There are eight levels of food, from pureed to chopped, with varying degrees in between.

Alpha House has forty residents in all, with a staff of three LPN's and one RN. Health workers are on probation for one year. The burnout rate is high. An organization called Green Lamps provides the foster grandparents. Kay Smith, the director of the unit, has had to fire only one foster grandparent (who was afraid to touch the children to whom she was assigned). Since the children don't recognize their foster grandparents, the level of gratification must be limited.

Professional staff members, as well as foster grandparents, must attend an annual conference on each resident. Team meetings must be called in the interim if a resident hasn't shown training progress within a three month period. Some residents in Alpha who are not making progress will go to another building for what has been recently dubbed "Foundation Care." Hampton Carmine had already introduced me to the term. Foundation Care, offered in another facility, concentrates simply on nurturance. Less task-oriented, less concerned with reporting progress, Foundation Care reduces the amount of documentation required and no longer treats "stimulation" as the ideal. "They get stimulation coming out of their ears." "Maybe what they really need," Smith said, "is just to be held."

Miscellaneous notes in the course of the day tended to support Carmine's and Smith's views. Some occupational training should be renamed and justified not as "occupational" but rather as training in elementary levels of self-care. Indeed, in some cases the procedure trains the trainer more than the resident. For example, a staff member who works with a patient having difficulty swallowing food learns how to present the food correctly on the tongue, to be patient before introducing more food, and to massage the throat in order to help it down. Such therapy, of course, has nothing to do with preparing a resident for a job. Or again, a staff member will introduce a pencillike cylinder between a patient's clenched finger, not so much to help the patient learn how to hold an object, but simply to create enough space in the clenched finger to air it out and reduce the smell of corrupting skin. Toilet training, in some cases, doesn't mean bringing the resident to the point that he or she can manage the task unassisted or even signal a staff member of imminent need; it simply establishes a chart showing times at which what most parents call "accidents" occur and therefore enables a staff member to get the resident to the toilet on time.

Two theories of care contended with one another at Caswell: one was more active and aggressive, pointed toward achievement; the other was more nurturant and affirming of the resident as he or she is.

In a sense, this conflict reflects, on a huge institutional scale, the tensions I found earlier in the testimony of parents who have reared retarded children under their own roofs, or, indeed, the tensions that anyone faces in dealing with someone to whom love binds him. Bonding generates a deep loyalty to both the being and the well-being of another. Human love and institutional care also require both; each loyalty is defective without the other.

If one settles for a simple affirmation of the being of another, just as he is, without attempting to enhance his capacities, love is quietistic; it may even slacken into the sentimental, or slide over into neglect. The object of love, even though treasured, lapses into little more than a collectible in a drawer or bin. But if one orients to the well-being of the other, to the enhancement of his capacities, to his measurable performance, then one begins to badger him or even to resent him as he is. That is the message from Hampton Carmine and Kay Smith. Institutional care for the retarded requires loyalty to both their being and their well-being. Administrators, professionals, and staff workers, at their best, work somewhere poised between the two.

Other visitors spent time in the residence hall that housed aggressive residents. Their visit led to table talk with Val Carmine about "aversive" training. Staff members are not permitted to strike or punish residents. They can resort to other modes of "aversive control" only when "positive reinforcement" doesn't work. She cited a case of aggressive self-abuse in which a resident struck the lower half of her face a thousand times a day and reduced the flesh on her jaw to a pulp. Staff had to resort to a spray can that squirted warm water into her eyes to keep her from hitting herself. But eventually the resident "manipulated" the procedure by bringing the spray can to the attendant whenever she wanted to beat her face. She recognized the spray can as a part of the total procedure. As a last resort, and upon approval of authorities, a staff member can pass ammonia under a resident's nose to divert from abusive behavior.

Val Carmine and Mary Lingerfelt-Heckrotte ran an evening session on Preventive Intervention Techniques (PITS), a set of purely defensive wrestling holds they teach attendants to use when dealing with residents who threaten to injure themselves or others. The techniques help staff members ward off blows and break holds without injuring the aggressor. Carmine and Heckrotte also demonstrated how to place the aggressor in "hands-on" restraints, positioning the attendant behind the back of the resident, holding the resident's left wrist with the attendant's right hand and the right wrist with the left hand. The resident's arms, thus pulled down and across in front of him, create a kind of self-enveloping straitjacket. Caswell Center prohibits altogether the use of mechanical restraints—straitjackets and the like. A hands-on restraint is personal; a straitjacket is impersonal, isolating, and more likely to be relied on for too long a time. For the same reason, Caswell urges restraining by hand the temporarily violent patient rather than locking him up in a room. If you lock him up, you are likely to forget about him; not so, if you are holding him yourself.

The women obviously enjoyed putting on the show. They have taken it on the road, so to speak, to service clubs and the like. They are good actors and athletes, with an instinctive sense for play that marks the exceptional language teacher, swimming coach, or trainer.

Their demonstration makes a point that students in a seminar on applied ethics might well take in. These staff members faced a classic conflict between goods of end (health and safety) and a good of process (personal freedom). For the sake of the end (the safety of the resident and third parties), staff members needed to curtail liberty. The need to limit liberty in a particular instance, however, should not allow the goods of process to vanish or evaporate; the goods of process ought to maintain a pressure upon one in the pursuit of the goal.

The staff members' "road show" also points the way for students who giddily rebound from a naive absolutism to an equally naive relativism. Once students discover that no given good is absolute, they assume that all is awash in the sea of the relative. They do not pay attention to the way in which a given good, even though limited, should maintain its pressure upon the sensitive agent as he or she pursues a more urgent goal.

Specifically, one ought to make sure that the goal is important and urgent, that it can be reached only by the limitation, and that the limitation should be as minimal as possible, for as short a time as possible, and with as few adverse consequences upon the person who must suffer the limitation. These criteria argue for wrestling handholds rather than mechanical restraints.

The women's technique supplies a parable for the humane administration of total institutions and, even more broadly, for the balancing of liberties and goods in a nation. The tyrant, as opposed to the humane political leader, for example, invokes emergency restrictions and powers when less severe measures might do as well to reach a national goal, fails to declare the emergency over as soon as he should or could, and either recklessly or punitively fails to keep to a minimum the injurious impact of the limitations upon those who suffer them. Just possibly, the women's wrestling techniques also supply us with a parable for the superiority of small-group facilities over huge institutions in delivering care to some of the retarded. A society should meet the needs of the retarded in the least restrictive way possible and also in ways that let members of the society learn how to touch, "hands-on," as it were, some of its own.

THE GESTATED
AND SOLD

MANY MEDICAL ORDEALS have resulted from advances in medical technology that have occurred without corresponding advances in our abilities to deal with the long-term results of applying that technology. In such "hard cases," the principal actors pay a huge price in suffering —Dax Cowart, Karen Quinlan's parents, the principals in the Elizabeth Bouvia case and in the Baby Doe, Baby Fae, and Baby M cases, and the like. We call these *hard* cases, but we get inured to that term. "Hard" means that no matter which way people turn, they suffer. However they decide, they face numbness and tragedy. Moreover, the often intrusive attention which the media,[1] educators, and professional conferences impose compounds the tragedy. People who never expected or wanted celebrity suddenly find themselves isolated, spotlighted, and publicly tried in the media. They suffer all the indignities of a simultaneous public trial, carnival, and soap opera. Yet such cases raise important issues in public policy that require us to review and clarify our understanding of civilized life and, in this present case, to illuminate the generative and providential tasks of parenting upon which that life depends.

Dr. William Stern paid $20,000, half to a fertility center and the other half to Mary Beth Whitehead, who agreed to be artificially inseminated with sperm from Dr. Stern and to carry to term a baby, which Mrs. Whitehead would then turn over to Dr. Stern and his wife, Dr. Elizabeth Stern, to rear as their own. Mrs. Whitehead changed her mind and wanted the baby back. But, as a lawyer friend of mine put it, "A deal's a deal." The judge in the trial court in New Jersey awarded custody of the now famous Baby M to the baby's biological father.[2] Judge Harvey R. Sorkow denied visiting rights to Mary Beth Whitehead, and, "immediately after reading his decision to the press, . . . called the Sterns into his chambers so that Mrs. Stern could legally adopt the child."[3]

Let me concede two propositions at the outset on the issues raised by the Baby M case:

1) The problem of infertility ought to command our sympathy. A couple desiring to have a child touches us more than does a couple that thinks only about its stocks or the new house or car it wants to buy. We can be grateful that *in vitro* fertilization and other techniques help some infertile couples to have children. We can be glad that adoption agencies permit still others to take on the responsibilities of parenting.

2) The marketplace is a valuable mechanism for distributing money, merchandise, and services. It lets us exchange work for money and buy a huge variety of goods and services that gratify wants and needs. A society without a free marketplace rests upon command and obedience alone. It lacks dexterity; it is all thumbs. The marketplace is a splendid specialized mechanism in its place and sphere.

But, at the same time, the market's place and sphere is, and should be, limited. We do not believe that the market should sell everything. We live in different spheres, and different principles of distribution apply in different spheres. We do not believe, for example, that we should sell judges' decrees. We forbid the bribery of judges and juries because payoffs corrupt the very meaning of justice, which should be impartial, blind, unmoved by the sweet talk of money. We also do not believe that money should buy exemptions from the burden of military service in war. In the Civil War, some rich men bought commissions, and others hired poor men to fight for them. We blocked that sort of activity in World Wars I and II, but we slipped sideways into the practice in the Vietnam War, as disproportionate numbers of the poor, who could not pay for college exemptions, ended up with their names engraved on Bangladesh marble near the Lincoln Memorial. We believe further that we should not sell grades in school or prizes at sporting events and in artistic or intellectual competitions. We would corrupt the very substance and meaning of these awards and honors if we sold them on the open market to the highest bidder.

We also shy at letting a person sell body parts—an eye or a kidney —to another. A society demeans itself and its members and fails to solve its problems fittingly if it exploits the penurious to sell a part of themselves. The rich ought not solve their health care needs through the desperation of the poor.

Similarly we have thought it a bad idea to give the family *full* property rights in the body of a deceased member. The family has *quasi* property rights, in the sense that the responsibility to provide fitting and appropriate burial falls upon the family; but it cannot *sell* body parts or auction off a particularly notorious dead relative to the highest bidder—to a carnival, or to some other institution with a profit opportunity in mind.

The same restriction on the marketplace applies to adopting babies. We do not think it right to sell or auction infants or children as products or commodities.

In sum, what we have marked out here are a few of the territorial limits of the marketplace and the contractual exchanges upon which it depends. Michael Walzer calls these boundary points "blocked exchanges," beyond which one corrupts, demeans, and distorts the good exchanged or acquired.[4]

In my judgment, the Baby M case ought to belong to one of these blocked exchanges. We misinterpret and corrupt the meaning of bearing and parenting a child when we pull them into the arena of a commercial transaction. And make no mistake about it: surrogate brokering grew into a substantial business. The *New York Times* on June 26, 1988 quoted Noel P. Keane, the lawyer who matched and arranged the contract between William Stern and Mary Beth Whitehead, as saying of his Infertility Center of New York, "We've had 238 children born, with 40 more on the way." His statement implies that his infertility center made some $2.5 million at $10,000 per transaction.

Judge Sorkow did seek to distinguish the Stern/Whitehead controversy from straightforward commerce in babies. First, he sought to decide in the "best interests of the child," the usual standard in an adoption or divorce proceeding. This attempt suggests that he would not simply decide the case on the evidence of money changing hands. He would assess the Sterns and the Whiteheads, to see which parents would provide the better home for the child. The judge conceded that Dr. Elizabeth Stern, a pediatrician, had, without benefit of outside professional judgment, diagnosed herself as suffering from multiple sclerosis, which she determined to be a risk to her in bearing a child. She also had not sought out professional help to determine the implications of this condition for a pregnancy, and she had misrepresented her infertility. But Judge Sorkow found the Sterns, on the whole, to be "credible, sincere, and truthful people," whereas Mrs. Whitehead's behavior had convinced him that she had a "fundamental inability to speak the truth."[5] He concluded that the Sterns would make better parents than would the Whiteheads.

Some critics have argued that the rhetoric of the judge's appraisal (and that of court psychiatrists) reflected a marketplace bias in favor of the rich and a class bias in favor of professionals who know how to talk to other professionals, and against an agonized working-class mother who did not know how to behave plausibly toward lawyers, judges, and psychiatrists.

The New Jersey Supreme Court review of the case did not entirely agree with this criticism of the judge's decision. The court allowed custody of the child to remain with the father, since the evidence "clearly proved such custody to be in the best interests of the infant," but in other major particulars the court reversed the trial judge's decision. It found "the payment of money to a 'surrogate' mother illegal, perhaps criminal, and potentially degrading to women" and therefore voided "both the termination of the surrogate mother's parental rights and the adoption of the child by the wife/stepparent" and restored the "'surrogate' as the mother of the child. . . ."[6]

The state supreme court foresaw deeper issues in the precedent-setting features of this case. A court can easily condone a rescue operation to save one specific child. It is quite another matter to issue a decision that will enter the literature and establish precedent for future cases in a form that would let a woman sell her right to control her health care in the course of a pregnancy, that would effectively consign to another person decisions as to whether to abort or to carry to term a fetus, and that would regularize and normalize the commercial practice of surrogate motherhood. The further reason Judge Sorkow gave for his original decision carries particularly troubling consequences.

Judge Sorkow had a problem which he solved dubiously. His first reason (deciding in the child's "best interest") pulled the Baby M case toward the jurisdiction of family law governing adoption. That body of law allows a judge to decide a case on the basis of the "best interest" of the baby. But adoption law also prohibits selling babies. Judge Sorkow therefore had to pull the case out of the orbit of adoption law, since the Sterns paid $10,000 to Mrs. Whitehead and $10,000 to a lawyer-broker in the case. Sorkow's solution? He distinguished between a service and a product. William Stern was hiring Mrs. Whitehead to carry the baby, he was not buying the baby from her. The court could not charge him with buying the baby, because genetically he already owned the baby. Thus, Sorkow concluded, the transaction did not reduce the baby to a commodity. Stern bought only the services of the biological mother, not the product of those services. The product was already his.

Now, the actual terms of the contract make it clear that the judge's distinction flies in the face of the facts. The contract oriented relentlessly to the product, not the process. If the mother lost the child through a miscarriage before the fifth month of pregnancy, William Stern would pay her nothing; if she had a stillbirth, Dr. Stern would owe her only $1,000, not the $10,000. The full $10,000, in this one-sided contract and others like it, lies in escrow until the mother delivers the baby to its owner. Clearly the contract requires delivering a product. And when the mother delivers that child, the contract requires that she relinquish her rights as its genetic mother, her presumptive rights of custody over an already extant child. It is baby selling.

In addition to this *bad faith* in his reasoning, that is, the judge's pretense that the contract did not enforce a sale, his very distinction between a service performed and a product distorts the human meaning of giving birth to a child. This distinction reduces parenting to *manufacturing*. In manufacturing, we correctly distinguish between the process and the product of that process. Ordinarily, workers don't develop deep ties to the monkey wrenches or to the sump pumps they produce. It would be bad if they did. Sales would suffer: workers make products in order to sell them. Workers can take pride in their products, but they had better not agglutinate to them, or their company is in deep trouble. Indeed, they've got a problem if they don't move the product beyond the loading dock. An older language called workers "alienable" from the fruits of their labor. Producers of commodities hire marketers, experts in figuring out how to move the product into alien hands. Our alienable relations to things differ from our inalienable rights and the inalienable rights of children, by which I mean rights we cannot sell without assaulting and demeaning their and our innermost identities.

The judge clearly used the metaphor of manufacturing in settling the case. He discerned a clear-cut distinction between the service of processing a baby and the baby as a product. He assumes that the law can tidily separate the two. Dr. Stern pays for the process, not the product. Sorkow's metaphor reduces the woman's irreversible sale of her maternal rights to her child to a minor, easily negotiated detail.

The metaphor of manufacturing doesn't help in interpreting carrying and bearing a child. To detach that *process* from the child who emerges from the womb and to assume that one can sell the first without the sale affecting the second advances male obtuseness to a new height. Justice should be blind, but not stupid.

The metaphor of manufacturing overlooks altogether the reality of human bonding. We bond intensively. As indicated in the chapter on the retarded child, human beings biologically depend upon bonding between the parents and the young to a degree that other animals do not. The opossum clings to the body of its mother, but the human baby cannot. It depends upon its mother to hold it. It needs the mother's active cradling, holding, cherishing, begun in the womb and carried forward into life for a time, and with an intensity unknown to any other creature. Human society depends heavily on the success of that bonding at every level from the womb through the wayward adventures of the child's education.

I would not want to claim that humans invariably bond. The substantial numbers of abortions and adoptions and the willingness of some women to put up their babies for sale prove the existence of many exceptions. These exceptions have persuaded the courts not to force a woman to carry a pregnancy to term or to keep and nurture a baby against her will. But at the same time, the propensity to bond works so powerfully that we call bonding not only usual but normal—so natural, indeed, that the state's enforcement of a commercial contract against Mrs. Whitehead's reconsidered wishes after bonding seems violent, not judicial.

These considerations lead me to oppose the type of proposal before the State Legislature of New York which would merely reform and regulate commercial contracts as they apply to surrogate motherhood, not eliminate them.[7] In particular, the legislature would require more fully developed informed consent on the part of both parties. (For example, the broker/lawyer in the Stern/Whitehead case hired psychiatrists to examine Mary Beth Whitehead. They reported to the broker/lawyer that she would probably not go through with the contract, but apparently the broker chose to withhold this information from Mrs. Whitehead and the Sterns. If the facts bear out this charge, the lawyer committed an appalling violation of his duties to clients: he withheld information crucial to them both in order to clinch the sale.) Second, the New York state law would insist on a prior court review to preclude such one-sided contracts as the Stern/Whitehead agreement.

This proposal to reform a commercial transaction does not go to the heart of the problem, however. To look at bearing a child as subject to a commercial contract distorts the event altogether. We should not regularize into law the separation of the genetic, gestational, and rearing tasks of parents except in rescue—that is, in adoption.

The alternative extreme of legislatively prohibiting surrogate motherhood creates a further set of difficulties, however. The state would find the prohibition difficult to enforce. Further, a law that criminalized the behavior of the mother, among other parties to a contract, might place the state in the awkward position of legislatively enforcing the natural human bonding between a mother and child by sending the mother to jail. Finally, an outright legislative prohibition of surrogacy might violate the constitutional right of privacy.

The Supreme Court of New Jersey has arrived at a more sensible solution to surrogate motherhood: it would not altogether prohibit such agreements, but, as it does in adoption, it would prohibit buying and selling children. A woman might still act as a surrogate mother, but not for hire. The law and the courts would discourage its commercialization in two ways: (1) by prohibiting the payment of a finder's fee, etc., to a third party, and (2), if money has changed hands between the two parties, by refusing to consider any contract or agreement legally enforceable. The full power of the state would not bear down to force the mother to give up her child, which is tantamount to saying that the exchange would come down once again to a gift. She would give the child as a gift, as she does in adoption.

Advocates of surrogate mothering argue that this policy would effectively eliminate the practice. It would knock out the commercial opportunity for a third party, with his prepared list of breeders, complete with pictures, psychological profiles, and IQ scores for each. Right and good! This elimination of a commercially interested third party might have the advantage of keeping legislation within the right-of-privacy clause of the U.S. Constitution, as the Supreme Court interprets it, while not denying altogether that special circumstances, which we cannot wholly anticipate, might make surrogacy defensible as a gift.

A member of the U.S. Congress drew an important boundary line recently when he said, "we want jurisdiction over the moneychangers in the temple; we do not want jurisdiction over the temple itself." The first part of his statement nicely marks out the territorial limits of the marketplace; the second, the equally important territorial limits of the state. As Samuel Johnson put the latter limits:

> How small of all that human hearts endure,
> That part which laws or kings can cause or cure.[8]

The state must both protect citizens against the marketplace but also, through its own self-restraint, respect the principle of the extraterritoriality of the person.

Undoubtedly, the Baby M case and others like it require public discussion as the society decides where it must draw its lines legally and morally. Surrogate motherhood is but one of many issues which advances in reproductive technology will pose for us. Increasingly, we will be tempted to reduce parenting to manufacturing. The term itself, "genetic engineering," speeds us along that road. Both negative eugenics, the art of eliminating deleterious genes and traits, and positive eugenics, the art of enhancing positive traits and capacities, tempt with the possibility of producing "designer genes." The agendas of negative and positive eugenics received a temporary setback when the Nazis embraced their goals in the 1930s. But in the next millennium, not unsavory totalitarians, but players in the marketplace will much more likely move us further in that direction. Fortunes will be there for the making by medical entrepreneurs who can grant the wishes of customers for superior children.

Few will deny the moral legitimacy of a disciplined negative eugenics that may help genetically blighted parents bear normal babies and thereby spare both parents and their children appalling ordeals. But the agenda of positive eugenics (enhancing memory, IQ scores, aggressiveness, and the like) would increasingly convert parenting into manufacturing. Moralist Francis Kane poses the long-range question: "Can anyone guarantee producing children according to our patent designs will be an act of self-giving love rather than vain self-display?"[9]

Clearly, we will not leave ourselves moral space for dealing with Kane's question if we discuss cases like Baby M in a form that distances ourselves from the behaviors scrutinized. As we play the roles of spectator and critic, we may fail to note our own subtle involvement in the behaviors examined and thus fail to prepare for the temptations ahead.

In these comments, for example, I have criticized the Baby M contract and the original judicial decision that supported it for treating a child as a product. But the temptation to treat a child as a product does not simply beset only the childless couple such as the Sterns or the judge who sides with them. Many parents yield to the temptation to treat their children as products when they live out their lives vicariously through the performance of their children. By midlife, parents see only too clearly the limits of their own lives, and they often press their children to conform to the idealized image of what the parents believe their child ought to become. They measure the child's performance against that image and signal rejection to the child when the child fails to live up to that standard or lives up to a different standard. Parents gradually slip into thinking like a manufacturer or an engineer. They become relentlessly product-oriented.

Parents may need to recognize that marriage and parenting resemble dirt-farming more than engineering. Shakespeare once put it, crudely, "Caesar ploughed her and she cropped." In the changing seasons of married and family life, one turns the soil, broadcasts a little seed, prays for a little sun and rain, and hopes for the best.

Perhaps, then, the Baby M case delivers a message to all of us beyond the harsh judgments heaped on the deafened and beleaguered Sterns, Whitehead, and Judge Sorkow.

Parenting (even that sly parenting that mates furnish one another) includes two demands always in some tension with one another. On the one hand, parents need to affirm the *being* of the child; they need to accept the other as he is. As Frost said, home is where they have to take you in. Parenting requires accepting love. On the other hand, parents must also encourage and foster the *well-being* of the other, the child. They must promote the child's excellence. If they merely accept the other as he is, they may neglect the important business of his full growth and flourishing. Parenting requires transforming love.

Clearly, perhaps especially in a meritocratic society, we have tended one-sidedly toward transforming. We have fiercely demanded performance, accomplishment, and results. At our worst, we drive our ambition through our children like a stake through the heart. We behave like the ancient Gnostics who despised the given world. We reject the child for flawed achievements. We fall into the traps set by a society that insists on accomplishment in payment for acceptance. We increasingly define and seize upon our children as products. Medical technology simply enabled and lured the Sterns and Mary Beth Whitehead into acting out the parental assumptions of a one-sided modern culture. There, out in the open, in the glare of the klieg lights, the principals found themselves faced with a public ordeal. But, in the reflected light of that public ordeal, the double ordeal in all one-sided parenting was exposed.

Parents find it difficult to maintain an equilibrium between the two kinds of love. Accepting love, without transforming love, slides into indulgence and finally neglect. Transforming love, without accepting love, badgers and finally rejects. No wonder, then, that parenting leads so often to a sense of defeat—unless, in the divine comedy of things, parents discern an equilibrium of a different order, a transcendent parenting that embraces both their children and themselves in all their imperfections. This transcendent equilibrium goes by the name of justifying and sanctifying grace. God forgives but also empowers; God affirms but also transforms. That is the good news for parents behind the judgmental news that besets the Sterns and Whitehead and haunts us all.

THE BATTERED

A SUPPORT GROUP of battered women met for their last session together. They did not all gather at 6:00 P.M., as planned, for their graduation ceremony. One woman sat alone, smoking. A staff member introduced us—first names only—and left.

I worried about being there. Under the best of circumstances a stranger disturbs the rhythm and tone of talk between friends. A battered woman might find a stranger even more intrusive. I had heard about the battered woman's isolation, her long-held secret, her fear of the outsider, her need to cover and protect.[1]

But she said she didn't care if I used her name and told her story to everyone who would listen. More people ought to know how some women lived, had to live, because the man had you under his control six different ways. And the legal system didn't help. Four years ago she had left him for a shelter. Last fall she got him out of the house, and, though she still dated him, she hoped for a divorce. Why did they date? Well, partly because she loved him. That was true. He also claimed that he had learned something, the time she finally decided to separate from him. But that was bullshit. The pattern was there. His first wife left him within six months of their marriage and the second left him after thirteen years of marriage.

Didn't you walk into this knowing, to some degree, what you were getting into?

Yes, but his second wife was a bitch. I'll give him that.

You thought his second wife might have deserved a beating? It would be different for you?

Yeah. But now I know better. He's done it always. His mother beat him when he was a kid, and that's the way he does it with me, to keep me under control, not just to keep me from stepping out of line, but to keep me in place. There's a difference. I'm talking about jail. That's what a jail is, keeping you in place.

Don't just say I love him and that's what keeps me with him. I have tried and I am trying to divorce him. But that takes six hundred dollars for the lawyer's fee and I haven't got it. If the house sold, I'd have it. He's agreed to sell the house, but he won't sign it over to me now to let me be free to sell it. So I need his cooperation until I've got a buyer.

That's one reason I date him. He'd get mad at me if I didn't. He tore up the house so badly on one rampage that I couldn't begin to sell it without repairs. Right now, I've got it down to the point that just a few hundred dollars would fix it up enough to show it for sale.

But that money doesn't come easily. I used to make three thousand a month, and even more, but my firm wouldn't put up with all the mess and turmoil of the marriage. I had to take time off—more time than the company would allow—when my husband beat me up or when he tore up the house. My field of work is a small world. Word gets around fast. I'm blackballed the way things are now. At most, I can make only eight hundred dollars a month now.

Another woman, arriving late, picked up on the point, the trap that keeps a woman locked in: A couple of years of crisis and your work record suffers; too many interruptions mess it up—the arrival of the police, visits to the hospital, the house torn up, arrangements made to fix it up, and the need to ship out the kids to protect them. Soon you begin to bounce from job to job. The record looks even worse. You can only get loser's jobs, and you end up less able to finance a divorce and support your kids.

So time is your enemy. When you come into the hospital and they see you beat up and the policeman sees your face, he's willing to testify, he's on your side. That's when they would be willing to do something, to put him in jail, to get going on the divorce. But if you punt then, everything gets harder. The legal system works against you. Everything takes time. They tell you they've got all the papers, but the day of the court hearing comes and they are missing an affidavit, so they put everything off—even though you asked them just before the hearing whether they had everything and you would have been glad to get whatever they're missing. So you wait, and all that waiting weakens your position—on starting a regular life, on landing something other than a loser job, on getting his cooperation on the sale of a house, or the motorcycle, or whatever, to keep things going. So the delays in the legal system give him all sorts of leverage, which makes you think, what's the use, why not punt? And because they think you're going to punt anyway, they see no reason not to slow things down.

Constables make no effort to find husbands to serve papers on them: One time they left the papers with his mother! That did no good. He has to get them directly. But try to find him. Now that he's out of the house, he moves around. Even when I know where he is and tell them, they still manage to be too late to nail him. Meanwhile, he still comes around the house, and I love him, despite everything, and he gets mad if I date anyone else. Though I'll still do that. That's my business.

Three of the five women said that liquor figured in their husbands' problems: They hit when they are drunk. But they aren't so drunk that, when they smash things, they smash their own stuff. They are sober enough to know how to go after you by trashing your things, what meant something to you.

The first woman emphasized that liquor didn't figure in her case: He's cold sober. He simply has to control my life in every detail. And everything seems to help him out—my drop in pay, the legal situation, and the slump in the real estate market. So you end up feeling that the whole world smells out weakness and moves in.

It's not difficult to tell someone who is battered. You can tell. It shows on their faces. Bruises heal, but the face changes in time. We can look at someone and know that she has a problem, even if bruises no longer show. There's a mark on her that shows no matter what you do.

Battering bruises not only the body but the soul. The battered sends out signals to the predator, the one who knows how to exploit. As one woman put it: He finds you out. Batterers are all alike. We have talked about it a lot. The men we deal with resemble one another over and over again.

A woman silent to that point declared that once free, she doesn't plan to get involved with a man ever again. She's had it. Not all were sure. The woman who had dogged the law courts said that one of the policemen at the emergency room, who tried to talk her into pressing charges immediately, has since dropped by a time or two. Others have helped: A friend, when she saw me, got out her camera and took pictures to make sure that we had some evidence. She also made me go down to the emergency room to create a record there and to secure witnesses. I don't know where I'd be if she hadn't made me do that. It's amazing how the thing fades for others. Somehow a family squabble doesn't seem to interest the state. We don't get equal protection from the law. If my husband did to another man at work what he's done to me, the cops would be on him fast. The law wouldn't tolerate it.

But his wife and children seem to be his property. At home, he can do what he wants.

I asked whether the men abused anyone and everybody, in private and in public. One woman said, he's just mean, period. But most saw the pattern of the bully, who smells out the weak. He abuses only those who can't hit back and only when no one stronger can intervene. The most verbal of the four spoke appreciatively of her boss who has stood by her, thus sparing her the need to drift down to a loser job. When, for example, she began to receive anonymous, hang-up phone calls, he picked up the phone and called her husband by name and told him if he didn't stop, he would come after him personally. The phone calls promptly stopped. And then, there's that policeman who has stopped by a time or two: "Who knows," she said. "Do you think I may, at last, have met Mr. Right?"

THE SCOPE, CHAIN, STRUCTURE, AND TEMPO OF VIOLENCE

Violence includes any and all force that invades, twists, flouts, distorts, injures, degrades, or crushes the victim. Physical force defiles. Even when innocent, the victim feels guilty and tainted. The violence has altered one's innermost being. One inexpungibly has to accept into one's being what one did not invite or provoke. Theft and plunder palely resemble rape. The thief forces into the sanctuary. He steals goods, trashes others. He violates and stains the house. Things never look the same again. The intruder has done more than steal; he has permanently weakened this place of safety and sanctuary, smeared it with the potential of his return. The eruption of violence between a man and a woman similarly trashes the core of her identity. However pacific the intervals between beatings, the woman knows that the man can break in at will. Suffering personal violence shames the victim. The violated does not simply suffer a bruised shin or a broken bone. Violence batters her core identity. The beating, even though temporary, stains and lowers self-esteem.

Violence comes in three forms: episodic, chronic, and institutional.

Episodic physical violence breaks out suddenly, disrupting life's apparently peaceful rhythms. Newspapers sell this sort of violence. The statistics boggle the imagination. In Texas:

—370,207 women suffered from spouse abuse in 1986.[2]
—Victims supply some hospital emergency rooms with 20 percent of their business.[3]

—A boyfriend or friend kills one of four murder victims.[4]

—Battering causes one quarter of all attempts at suicide by women.[5]

In the USA:

—*Time* magazine reported, using figures from the National Council on Domestic Violence, that six million women suffer physical abuse each year.[6]

Chronic violence, less obvious but no less deadly and distorting than episodic violence, shows up in the form of what we euphemistically refer to as stress and pressure. When we say he or she was under pressure, we refer to a relentless pounding on the psyche that deforms the core of one's being, one's regulating capacities, one's command and control. Episodic violence often erupts out of stress. The apparently peaceful, unobtrusive, quietly cooperative neighbor suddenly blows up and kills wholesale. Chronic pressure can eventually crush a man's hold on himself, and when he lets go, he collapses or explodes.

Finally, violence includes what social analysts have lumped under "institutional violence": the slowness of the courts; chronic unemployment that affects 40 to 50 percent of a given minority's teenagers; the lack of adequate prenatal and postnatal care for pregnant teenagers and their often premature babies; and inadequate training for adopting parents and foster parents. These institutional affronts often take a passive rather than an active form, which cloaks them in invisibility. But the obdurate passivity of institutions, their unresponsiveness to fundamental human needs, and specifically to the needs of the victim, injures and blights futures. Indeed, discrete episodes of violence and violating pressures and structures forge a chain of violence that binds from generation to generation.

Violence breeds violence. The figures attest to the fecundity of violence from generation to generation. Sixty percent of men who batter and twenty percent of battered women grew up in battering homes. Eighty-five percent of men in prison grew up in such homes.[7] Current child abuse guarantees a generation of spouse abusers to come. In 1983, the Texas courts determined that almost 60,000 children in the state suffered from abuse or neglect. Abuse or neglect killed 120 children in 1982. Child services protect, more or less, a total of 123,500 children in Texas at any given time.[8] We can reasonably expect, if past patterns prevail, that large numbers of these children of violence will, as adults, batter their spouses and abuse their children. W. H. Auden once summarized this downward chain of violence in four compressed lines:

> For shameless Insecurity
> Prays for a boot to lick,
> And many a sore bottom finds
> A sorer one to kick.[9]

This chapter will concentrate on battering men and battered women. Not that the phenomenon of battering takes only this form. Women also batter men; men and women batter children (with the woeful results, just noted, from generation to generation); and older brothers and sisters batter their younger or less powerful siblings. I will concentrate on men battering women, since it provides the more typical pattern among adults; and the child suffering abuse will receive attention in the chapter on the molested. Perhaps this focus on the typical pattern will nevertheless yield some insights on the structure and rhythm of violence, its assaults on human identity, and available types of treatment which will apply more generally to other forms of domestic violence.

Structurally, family violence resembles those repetitious horror films that isolate, mutilate, and threaten to kill. The lord of the castle isolates the victim from the society at large in the space that he controls. There he exercises utterly disproportionate power over her. The walls are thick, the moat is wide, and the bridge drawn up. She experiences a terrible isolation, powerlessness, and helplessness; the lord of the castle controls all the levers of power.

But, in addition to these structural similarities to the trap set by the villain in the Gothic novel, the abused spouse can despair of the external world. The dilatory legal system arrives a day late and a dollar short. The economic system often effectively starves her back into "jail." Emotionally, moreover, she cannot easily escape a prison which—however oppressive, miserable, chaotic, and tightly controlled—she also knows as her home, the site of a one-time love. The home not only signifies oppression, misery, and traps, but also normalizes them into the only world she knows. Therefore she cannot see escape as pure rescue; escape also threatens to annihilate her world. Healing does not simply offer life and health but also forces her to kill and bury the past she at least partly loved. Ethicists underestimate the ordeal that people face in the moral life when they euphemistically refer to "trade-offs," as though people in trouble need only spread out, like accountants, a balance sheet. In fact, people in trouble resemble more voyagers and pioneers who, even while conflicted with grief and relief, seek to scramble ashore in an alien land.

Moralists also pay too little attention to the elements of rhythm and tempo in life and thus to the specific world that bears down upon a group of people. By cutting up life into discrete decisions, moralists neglect the great overarching rhythms of work and play, the tempos of life in the restaurant, the hospital, the city desk, the airport, the night club, the precinct station, the stock exchange, the jogging path, the highway, and the home that pulse through individuals and that make specific moves seem morally plausible. Outside those patterns, in another time and place, these decisions would lose their justifying beat. Moralists often neglect the myriad of details that surround behavior. Media and film directors, more than moralists, fully recognize and manipulate the urgent patterns of sound, movement, and color that provide us with our behavioral cues.

Rhythm leads us past conscious barriers and taboos into ecstasy. Social dancing relies on the invitation of rhythm to move people beyond the shyness that the conscious mind imposes. What thought might help us avoid doing in another time and place, familiar sounds and rhythms help us slip into reflexively. Religious ecstacies have sometimes rocketed into sexual recklessness fueled by handclapping, rhythmic shouting, and dancing. The tempo of production in the modern factory often creates an urgent beat that justifies neglect of such prosaic matters as workers' safety, environmental protection, and safe products. Such patterns of time and momentum do not excuse a particular action or moral offense any more than Nixon's men could excuse their behavior by their weak appeal to "at that point in time" or "in that time frame." But therapists and ethicists seriously underestimate the power of a given human problem if they neglect the importance of tempo and atmosphere in shaping it.

Family violence, the literature tells us, follows the rhythm and tempo of addiction. Violence and addiction link in two ways: first, addictive substances and drugs, chiefly alcohol, accompany violence in 60 to 80 percent of the cases; and second, the activity of beating itself can addict the bully and the bullied. Various addicts, analysts have often observed, not only fix on a substance (liquor, food, cigarettes, dice, or clothes) but also on the rituals they associate with the substance (drinking, eating, smoking, gambling, or flashing credit cards). The full-blown addict locks on the substance or activity partly out of desire and partly looking for relief from his frustration and fears. Since, in the course of time, a given dose fails to relieve, the addict often increases the dose or shortens the interval between takes. Toward the end, the addict's life narrows around the particular substance or activity. What used to offer him respite from his plight (or give him a sense of freedom by giving him power) becomes at length his jail.[10]

The batterer's behavior resembles that of other addicts, and not simply because alcohol or drug abuse often accompanies violence. The batterer resorts to violence as a junkie resorts to heroin. First, the hitter narcissistically logs a series of grievances, persuading himself that he suffers rather than gratuitously abuses. His needs alone have merit. He has shown her more patience than she deserves. But she keeps it up. She won't stop. Then the usual triggering incident, which, the first time, started violence almost by accident, now ignites him by reflex; it lets him flare up. "There she goes again. Didn't I warn her? This time, I'm really going to let her have it."

So he explodes into uncontrolled violence, without realizing that he has always been out of control. He has never governed himself.[11] Even the tight controls he imposes on her—the way he likes his food, the noise of the children to which he objects, the mistake he detests —all these controls flow from his uncontrollable fear that the world controls him. This fear provokes the final outpouring of his ecstatic rage; it lifts him out of his frightened state and gives him his perverted pentecost when he is "not himself!"

Afterwards, of course, he is able to write off the episode as a moment in which he was not himself. This ecstatic blankout makes it easier to repent, beg for forgiveness, and promise to amend—by which he means that he repents the episode, not his underlying character, with its correlative fear of the world, which remains intact.

Lenore Walker summarizes the pattern of violence by identifying its three phases:[12] (1) tension builds between the couple; (2) he batters; and (3) he apologizes and showers her with gifts and promises not to do it again. In the course of time, the tempo of violence picks up. (1) The cycle accelerates (the wheel moves from battering to battering in a month or less instead of a year); (2) the violence escalates; and (3) the respite shortens or altogether disappears (he does not even bother to express remorse; and tension builds soon after the last violent episode). The experienced counselor therefore tells the client at the close of an interview, "You can be sure of one thing: as bad as you think it is now, it will get worse."

What causes a sufficient break in the rhythm of violence to prompt the partners to seek therapy? Not often does the husband take the initiative. Of the one hundred men that one agency has seen, only one or two men have come in on their own. Many men make appointments only because a judge has ordered it, or because the man found an ultimatum attached to his pillow, or because the wife actually left or threatened convincingly to leave. Physicians at the municipal hospital refer patients to the agency, but they usually accept at face value the woman's explanation that she bumped into the cabinet door. Staff members at shelters feel they need to explain violence to physicians to help them recognize its victims. In 1988, the Surgeon General of the United States, Dr. C. Everett Koop, acknowledged that need and published an advisory to physicians to help them identify and treat the battered.

In some cases, an abused woman will not take steps until her spouse starts to hurt the children. When he crosses that boundary, the woman, who cannot bring herself to defend herself, will often defend her children. That not only attests to the power of a protective, maternal love, it also betrays some women's lack of self-esteem. The battered self no longer seems worth protecting. She accepts his brutality as the given world, the world to which she must yield without alternative. His good days and bad days are beyond her control. She can influence them as little as she can the weather, and she cannot leave him any more than a wheatfield can withdraw from a hailstorm. But damage to the child makes a clear-cut difference; it can prompt her more than any other factor to seek help.

Most of the research on abuse has emphasized its common features, its overarching pattern and the similarities between the men and women who participate in it. More recent research has emphasized the different patterns of abuse and the varying types of victims and victimizers. If the patterns of abuse and the participants differ, then, batterers and the battered may require different types of treatment.

One study, for example, of 119 women admitted to a Detroit shelter identified five types of abuse.[13] Type one consists of those couples who, except for relatively infrequent abuse, enjoy a stable relationship. Drinking often attends the abuse and the children are rarely abused. Women in such relationships were likely to remain with the spouse. Type two victims suffer a "highly unstable, explosive relationship with their assailant,"[14] who abuses them severely enough to injure them and often sexually. Women who fall into the third group suffer even more severe and chronic abuse, often accompanied by assaults on the children. Women so abused retaliate less often with violence of their own, but they are also the most likely eventually to leave their partners. Type four consists of women who are less likely to be married to their assailants. The woman suffers less abuse than her children. While she usually intends to return to her partner, in fact she is among the least likely to live with him after treatment. Type five includes women who have seen and suffered the most abuse or neglect in their families of origin and who have most resigned themselves to the violence that pervades their lives.

Different patterns of abuse, Snyder and Fruchtman and others have argued, justify different treatments. Behavior modification techniques, for example, work most effectively in interrupting the patterns of conflict that afflict couples in the first group. Women in the remaining groups, they believe, "require interventions aimed more directly at establishing independent arrangements."[15]

Other researchers have concentrated on patterns of personality and behavior among abusive men. After surveying those basic patterns already identified in the literature, Edward Gondolf uses a cluster analysis on a sample of 6,000 battered women admitted to shelters in Texas across an eighteen-month period.[16] He discerns three basic types of batterers: sociopathic (7 percent), antisocial (42 percent), and typical (51 percent). The first two types abuse severely and often, with the first group compiling an arrest record in crimes of violence, crimes against property, and drug or alcohol related crimes along the way. The "typical batterer," however, abuses the partner less, physically, verbally, and sexually, and the children less often and less severely. He conforms more often to the rhythmic pattern which Lenore Walker identified. His victim will more likely return to him after treatment.

Using the earlier work of Harry Stack Sullivan, as mediated through Silano Orieti's *The Intrapsychic Self*, therapist Sherry G. Lundberg of the North Dallas Family Place Help Center proposes a psychodynamic approach to domestic violence that views each case of male violence as individual rather than typical. Lundberg argues, on the basis of her case experience, that violent males react "to present situations 'as if' they were reliving the moment in terms of an earlier experience."[17] Specifically, "the cases all illustrate distorted reactions based on an abusive man's experience with his mother early in life."[18] The abuser acts out this earlier experience by battering his wife. This diagnosis centers on the patient's individual history and thus argues for individualized treatment. The counselor must help the patient attain insight into his personal history that will help break the thrall of the past and keep him from wrongfully and harmfully repeating "unfinished business."[19] One might question whether this approach sees cases as radically individual, since each batterer shares in common, however much the specifics of early history may differ, a tragic compulsion to repeat unfinished business with the mother. Suffice it to note that these differing interpretations of battering, batterers, and the battered push in different directions for treatment.

CHOICES IN TREATMENT

Therapists who deal with family violence face several basic questions in planning treatments with their clients. (1) Can or should the woman and her children move into a shelter and seek thereafter to live independently of the abuser? (2) Should the therapist use the methods of insight therapy, or of behavior modification? (3) Should the therapist work with individuals, with couples, or with groups segregated into victims and abusers? These three questions overlap; and therapists often, where appropriate, mix strategies.

The therapist who would remove the victim from the abuser's fists faces barriers both internal and external. The comments of battered women presented at the beginning of this chapter emphasize in detail those external barriers—attaining jobs, child care and schooling for the children, and finances—which discourage so many women. The external world often provides her with no safe haven; it batters just as surely, if not as conspicuously, as does the batterer.

Internal barriers exist as well. The woman—however much abused —may still love her husband. Even if anger and resentment engulf that love, she may feel psychologically unable to leave him. She cannot imagine herself functioning alone, for the world he forced on her has become the only world she knows. It defines her as worthy only of abuse, unfit for any other kind of life. Periodic beatings have deprived her of her sense of her body's integrity and, with that, her sense of personal dignity. Self-confidence depends upon body-confidence. When both go, the world senses it and stacks against victims. The person seems fit only for pushing around.

Sensing this state of affairs, the victim sticks with the world that she knows. She assumes that the larger, unknown world would only besiege her with more of the same, without, however, offering her the advantages of familiarity and the opportunities for petty manipulation that flow therefrom. Further, the familiar rhythm of violence may offer its own sad gratifications: the repeated build-ups of tension, the brutal outbursts, followed by the bittersweet reconciliations.

(One needs to be careful, however. The fact that the cycle of abuse offers some unconscious gratification to the abused and that she herself may become, at some level of her being, an addict does not exculpate the abuser. This addiction simply attests to the psychological scope of the abuse. The true victim does not remain inwardly free and untouched in the midst of outrage, but attunes herself to it. In her innermost being she begins to consent—as though there were no other terms and conditions for life and love. The woman who says "be it unto me according to thy word" simply exposes the depth of the abuse, she does not lessen the man's responsibility for it.)

The victim's double imprisonment in walls both external and internal resembles the control of organisms newly created by recombinant DNA. Scientists prevented the escape of these organisms into the external world in two ways: first, they contained them externally, by establishing isolation facilities and sterilizing zones, and, second, they contained them biologically, by building into the organisms a series of defects that prevent them from surviving outside the laboratory. If they escape, they die. Just so, the abuser not only isolates the victim, but, far more effectively, builds into her, over time, a series of psychological deficits that make it difficult for her to imagine herself surviving outside his psychological laboratory.

These external and internal barriers oblige counselors to offer two kinds of help: as advocates and as therapists. First, whether the client remains with her spouse or not, she will probably need temporary shelter, job training, skill in job interviewing, employment, welfare, child care, food stamps, legal aid, and help on schooling for her children. (The woman in the midst of a crisis who needs protection from her spouse can find the problem of schooling for her children particularly difficult. The aggressive spouse may attempt to locate her "safe house" by tracking the children home from school.) No matter how independent she may be as a person, she will need an advocate's help; some agencies will not see her without a professional validation of her need. This mobilizing of institutional resources may also indirectly help the woman psychologically. Knowledge of the existence of some resources gives her an edge even if she decides to return to her husband. Despite everything, she knows that some alternatives exist out there.

Further, the counselor needs to offer direct psychological help to the victim in coping with her own internal barriers to a reconstructed life. Thus the first decision the therapist and the client face—whether or not the client should leave the abuser—inevitably overlaps into the second and third—deciding on the most appropriate therapy and the setting for it.

Insight Therapy. Basically, therapists employ two methods for treating the parties to violence: insight therapy and behavior modification. Insight therapists see violence as a symptom and seek to get at its root. They try to trace it to roots in largely unconscious and longstanding conflicts within each party that play themselves out in their current destructive and self-destructive battles. To break reflexes and construct a future different from the past, therapists must help the patient go through a protracted and often painful revisiting of the past. Insight therapists are suspicious of shortcuts. Successful therapy must help create and release a new sense of the self and its plight to achieve any permanent change in external behavior. Insight therapists prefer to treat individuals or couples rather than large groups. They eschew working with large groups since the emphasis there falls on training rather than insight.

Some insight-oriented therapists also feel that they lessen the patient's chance for developing if they intervene directly in a crisis. They should not offer emergency help. They cannot act both as a flashlight into the psyche and as a chain saw cutting a firebreak against crisis. If the therapist forcefully intervenes, the client loses a sense of herself as responsible agent. The therapist changes into yet another actor (or director of the play), subject to all the ambiguities of action, interaction, and unforeseen consequence. Whether resented for her errors or, conversely, adored for her triumphs, the therapist reduces the patient to dependence, without abiding insight and confidence in herself. Thus the insight therapist must deliberately limit her actions. Emergencies may call for an interventionist, but that task she herself cannot undertake.

In addition to these self-imposed limitations, the approach of the insight therapist poses some practical difficulties for victims. It costs more, and it runs the danger of medicalizing the problem. Since insight therapy assumes long-term, usually one-on-one analysis, it costs more than any but the affluent can pay. If our society had to rely on this method alone, the vast majority of victims, usually poor, or cut off from their usual income, could expect little help. Further, in treating violence as a symptom, insight therapy tends to interpret the problem as medical rather than moral. However, regularly beating one's spouse not only indicates a sickness, it violates our morality. We cannot passingly interpret violence as a symptom that we hope one day will disappear. We must stop it immediately. This need argues for modifying behavior forthwith. (Strictly considered, of course, a medical interpretation does not demand that one ignore or defer treatment of symptoms. Medicos treat symptoms as well as and at the same time as they seek causes; they reduce the fever and give antibiotics.) In its basic agenda, however, insight therapy undertakes a more tortuous and prolonged exploration of the cognitive causes of violence.

That particular ordering of the agenda for treatment may fail to note that even modest successes in stopping bullying and beating may help one or both parties to see that they have a chance of changing their habits. Small victories may signify that the recurrent pattern of defeat that has darkened their lives need not endlessly prevail. For various reasons, then, therapists in the field today, including insight therapists, do not automatically assume that they must begin with insight in order to change or reduce symptoms. In fact, they will ask for changes in behavior as a condition of therapy. As one insight therapist put it, "I do not continue to work on the 'deeper issues' unless they stop the violence."

Behavior Modification. The behaviorally oriented authors of a workbook for violent men frankly begin with symptoms: "We say, 'stop the violence first,' then work on underlying pathology."[20] Profound transformations of identity and feeling, however impressive, may come too late to do either the abuser or the abused much good. Indeed, some modifiers hold that we cannot profoundly transform feeling. Anger wells up from midbrain activity that therapy cannot reach or change.[21] Nevertheless, therapy can train the patient to accept responsibility for his behavior, which, modifiers believe, lies within his capacity to change and control, despite the fiery intransigence of the midbrain and the admittedly addictive character of violent behavior.

The behavior modifiers deal less with the client's vision of the world and more directly with the rhythm of life which the vision helps create and which the client internalizes as habit—the habit of beating. The cyclical pattern in which the batterer lives destroys his mate and himself and at an accelerating pace. Thus to save both him and others, the therapist must break the external patterns that the batterer uses to justify his beating and the internal habits that control him, not by reconstructing a self psychoanalytically but by enforcing new habits and patterns of interaction.

To this end, therapists have devised a series of techniques to modify the abuser's and the victim's behavior. These techniques include the following:

1) The time-out. Therapists borrow from our more strenuous sports (and from the ancient practice of war) the convention of the time-out (the functional equivalent of the holiday in the traditional prosecution of war). When anger and tension build up, either party can call a truce. Both must go to neutral corners to cool off. The period lasts for an hour or longer. Since anger and fear increase body tension, exercise —such as a walk—helps both parties. The manuals warn against driving as too dangerous. They also urge ritualizing the signal for a time-out. The T-signal of the prize-fight ring will do or, even better, standard words such as "I'm beginning to feel angry. I need a time-out." Even though brief, the assertion itself packs in a lot. It makes a statement about the self; it asserts with "I," rather than accuses with "you." It confesses, moreover, the person's anger and need; neither confession comes naturally to the battering man. The partners should practice the time-out regularly, even when the situation does not call for it, as they would drill or exercise to improve skills in a sport. And they must agree to come back together again at some time and talk after calling a time-out.

2) Identifying and expressing feelings. Abusive men, on the whole, talk less well than their mates, acknowledge their feelings less well, and act on their anger rather than express it. Therapists thus tell clients to keep journals that record their incidents of anger and even estimate their intensity on a 1–10 scale. Sonkin and Durphy's handbook for abusive men[22] identifies three responses to anger: stuffing it (that is, repressing anger and therefore building up pressure toward the violent explosion); escalating it (that is, rushing headlong toward the explosion); and directing it. Only the third response offers a healthy solution. But in order to direct his anger, the abuser must also learn techniques associated with assertiveness training. (Sonkin and Durphy's insistence that battering men learn how to assert themselves violates common intuitions about treatment as much as does feeding amphetamines to hyperactive children.) Abusive men must learn how to say no and how to ask for what they want clearly and directly. Nonassertiveness leads to stuffing anger. Stuffing anger eventually leads to aggressiveness in other forms and escalates anger into rage. Only assertiveness offers the battered the chance to direct anger.

No one, of course, can direct anger too hot to handle. Thus the trainer teaches relaxation exercises to supplement the assertiveness training. Such exercises borrow heavily from the work of Dr. Herbert Benson[23] and others. The use of relaxation techniques may require theorists to enlarge their three-part analysis of the responses to anger. In addition to stuffing, escalating, and directing anger, batterers need to learn how to discharge the rage harmlessly into the ground, much as a dragging chain discharges the static electricity from a truck into the highway and prevents a fire or an explosion.

Jeanne Deschner's book on modifying violent behavior, *The Hitting Habit*,[24] urges training sessions on two further important techniques: "cognitive realignment" and "diplomatic intervention." The very title "cognitive realignment" suggests a salute in the direction of insight therapists. How can one seriously reshape habits if one does not offer a corrective vision of the world and the self to which the habits reflexively respond? The curricular training unit on cognitive realignment, however, employs a terse, assertional, autosuggestive mode, as the client tells himself or herself "This is no big deal, I can handle it." Such compact assertions reflect less cognition than faith. The abuser or the abused, despite all experience to the contrary (in which the self knew that it could not handle "it"), now *acts as if* the self controls itself, *as if* the irritants do not enrage. The abuser repeats the terse faith-statement in the hope that it will begin to change his world. While the technique may be useful, perhaps "cognitive realignment" misnames it. The invocation resembles rather the uttering of a mantra. The patient using it acts by faith rather than by sight.

The techniques of cognitive realignment rely, in effect, on the ancient stoic distinction between what lies within, as opposed to beyond, one's control and reassures the abuser that while he cannot control the irritating event, he can control his response to it. The abuser can repeat "It's no big deal, I can handle it" and thus teach himself to handle his attitude toward it. But sooner or later (unless he has acquired a stoic perspective and placed petty irritants in some cosmic context), he will want to change the behavior of his mate. He will want to submerge himself in the immediate and do something about all those annoyances that helped produce flare-ups in the first place. Assertiveness training itself will push him toward action. He will need some alternative to stoic resignation and uncontrolled rage.

At this point, behavior modification shifts from the techniques of cognitive realignment to those of diplomatic intervention. Assertiveness training now pushes the modified toward modifying the behavior of their partners. Unfortunately, the specific techniques recommended in diplomatic intervention expose behavior modification in its most dubious affronts to the intelligence and dignity of the abuser and the abused. For example, E. L. Phillips and colleagues[25] develop techniques for changing the spouse's behavior—diplomatically rather than confrontationally. While Phillips's exercises avoid the obvious errors of direct, blunt speech, they lapse into a style somewhat transparent, naive, managerial, and patronizing. Phillips offers the illustration and model of the husband who diplomatically corrects his wife (who has just burned the pork chops) with such lines as, "How about setting the timer when you put the meat in the broiler? Then you can do other things, even answer the phone, and dinner will still be perfect." This particular diplomat also offers her further positive reinforcements: "If you'll do that, I promise to fix the pot handle you wanted." After making good on this promise, he rewards her with the declaration, "Here is the pot, all repaired. I'm going to brag tomorrow at work about what a terrific cook you are." These lines should enrage the mildest of spouses and provoke her to pick up the repaired pot and apply it to the head of her in-house trainer.

While the manuals occasionally push the trainee toward an assertiveness that parodies the worst of the trainer's own techniques, one hardly finds grounds for dismissing the movement. Successful trainers usually work with groups, reinforce their training with individual therapy, and supplement it later by counseling the couple. Group work appeals to recently established, underfunded, and overcrowded social agencies for several reasons: it costs less than working with individuals; it helps clients overcome the terrors and shame of isolation; groups can help establish accountability and reinforce positive changes; and members can form individual friendships that outlast the group. The similarities in the plights of clients convince agencies that standardized techniques will solve their problems. Potential trainers who vary greatly in educational background can learn and use these explicit, defined, and simple training techniques. Thus the training handbooks read like high school workbooks and army manuals. The therapists at work in this newly expanding enterprise do not peddle boutique psychiatry.

We cannot yet definitively assess the effectiveness of behavior modification techniques. Although wife-beating and child-beating have long attracted moral criticism, not until recently has the public viewed them as a legitimate concern of the state. The results of insight therapy and behavior modification and the efforts of victims in support groups may take a decade to sort out, especially since conscientious therapists have aggressively and eclectically attempted to mobilize all possible resources and types of treatment for help.

However, behavior modification does provoke some skepticism, above and beyond the obvious dangers of its sometimes patronizing tone. In the first place, the philosophical determinism that helped give rise to its techniques fails to picture the universe in a way that would allow one to take both the picture-maker and the picture itself seriously (as true and not merely determined). The determinist, after all, hopes that we will accept his views as true and not simply as words that a wholly determined process forced him to utter.

Further, behavior modification assumes a psychological egoism in its strategies of negative and positive reinforcement. These strategies appeal frankly to self-interest. While trainers ought to appeal to self-interest, they may underestimate the capacity (and the need) of the most

morally bedraggled to expend themselves for others. Ironically, therapists expend themselves daily for clients in a measure and for reasons
that exceed psychologically and morally what the theory to which they
subscribe provides for. Behavior modifiers, of course, might deflect such
criticism by separating the techniques themselves from their philosophical background in determinism and psychological egoism. After all, not
too long ago Christian theologians concluded that they could shuck
Freud's reductionistic anthropology while retaining some of his insights
and his analytic techniques.

Gondolf and Russell[26] view behavior modification as positively dangerous or at least mischievous. The technique implies that the victim
provokes anger and precipitates abuse and that anger (rather than pre-
meditated behavior) causes abuse. It tempts the batterer to invoke anger
as an excuse and therefore encourages denial. Finally, its quick fix can
give victims the false impression that the batterer has the problem under
control and thus expose them to further danger. Such critics hold to
a more social/political interpretation of battering: ". . . wife abuse is
not necessarily anger-driven, but more the consequence of a socially
imposed 'need' to control women."[27] Thus they propose resocializing
men in the setting of theme-centered discussion programs that would
help "eliminate" sex-role stereotypes that contribute to men's tendency
to control women. This view sees abuse as part of a broader social pathology, a theory which in its own way risks supplying the abuser with
an excuse.

A final criticism of behavior modification returns us to the basic
reservation of the insight therapists: the technique concentrates on the
externals of behavior and neglects the internals—the client's vision of
himself and the world that rationalizes his violence. Amendment of life
depends upon correcting that vision. One cannot reconstruct one's future unless one has reinterpreted one's past and present. When people
act spitefully, vindictively, they do not usually do so in an existential
revolt against the universe they perceive. Rather, they believe that their
behavior suits that universe.

In the throes of abuse, abusers believe that the wife deserves what
she gets. She had it coming to her. A time-out would merely delay the
tempo of things, the action of physical law and metaphysical justice.
Interference from the outside—from social workers, police, and behavior modifiers—sabotages the just order of things the abuser upholds.
When the wife gets out of line, he must put her back in her place. When
the police and social workers invade the home, a domain not their own,
they also get out of line: they exceed their duties; they act unjustly.
This vision reflects the client's own experience. His parents often ruled
with the belt and the fist. A cycle of violence, like the cycle of the
weather, with its build-up of angry, humid clouds, its distant lightning,
its tornadoes, and its sunny stretches, rules his adult domestic life. His

picture of things reflects, he thinks, the cosmos itself and exposes any intervention as forced and illegitimate. No wonder that the male client often appears grudgingly in a therapeutic program and only because the courts have forced him to.

In response to these criticisms, particularly to the failure of behavior modification to generate insight and therefore modify the inner self, we need to distinguish between two ways of interpreting its techniques: restrictively or expansively. Restrictively considered, behavior modification does not pretend to change the soul, either because, in a sense, there is none (the view of the philosophical determinists) or because the inner self consists of a series of relatively intransigent neurological nexi (the midbrain reservoir of anger) which one cannot expect to eliminate or modify. Modifiers, so viewed, must content themselves with damage containment.

This more restrictive view of the purposes of behavior modification techniques resembles the conventional explanation given for the mechanisms and devices built into the Constitution of the United States. The founders of the Constitution and their chief apologists viewed human nature realistically, even Calvinistically. They knew that self-interest largely determined human life and that self-interested factionalism would tear the country apart unless they devised a method of government which balanced interest group against interest group and thus contained their negative and destructive effects. To that end, the founders designed several mechanisms (including the separation of powers and the division of governments into federal, state, and local), not to transform human nature, but simply to keep contentious human behavior within acceptable bounds. Given this limited sense of its task, a government could properly modify only the behavior, not the thought of its people. It could not constrain interior thought, speech, or religion.

Behavior modifiers set for themselves a very limited task, similarly conceived. They do not pretend to eliminate anger any more than the founders of the country felt that they could eliminate ravening self-interest from political life. Rather, through various techniques, they hope to keep anger within limits, to express it in an orderly way or to cool it, but, in any event, to avoid those dangerous repressions and escalations that savage equally the family and the Republic.

More expansively and perhaps ideally interpreted, behavior modification does not restrict itself to the externals of behavior. It begins, to be sure, with habits, but, eventually, it changes the psyche. Modified behavior eventually alters the client's perception of himself and his world. As one of the jingles of Alcoholics Anonymous puts it, just bring your body to the meeting and the mind will follow.

So viewed, behavior modification and insight therapy begin at opposite poles, but each tends toward the other. Insight therapy begins with the sick soul and hopes eventually to alter actions and habits.

Behavior modification begins by attempting to change actions and habits but, through that change, hopes eventually to reshape the self, to force it to see itself in a new perspective and possess itself in a new way.

The contrast between the American and the British traditions of acting offers an analogy for this second way of interpreting the differences between the two therapeutic approaches. On the one hand, the Stanislavskian or "Method" school of acting, exemplified and popularized in the United States by Marlon Brando, sought to break with the external conventions of the theater, the traditional artifices of the actor, and to achieve first an internal identity and fusion of the actor with the character he or she plays. The Stanislavskian actor must renounce the shortcuts of imitation and submerge his psyche within the inner history and aims of the character. Only later does he develop the gait, countenance, speech, and behavior that express that identity. Proceeding in that order the actor avoids, so the theory goes, the traps of automatized and stock performance.

Conversely, the British actor, in a more "presentational" tradition, begins with externals—the placement and timbre of the voice, the body's carriage, the choices of makeup and costume, walk and gesture —and, in the end, achieves and receives the character that fills in the form. Sir Laurence Olivier described this process as the way in which he worked up his Othello. He did not begin by searching for the inner Othello, but experimented first with voice placement, skin color, costume, and carriage to help him eventually reach that persona which the performance required.[28]

These two acting methods do not produce identical results, but neither method altogether rejects what the other affirms as its point of departure. The first works at inner identity and eventually receives the externals as gift and outcome. The second works at the externals first and eventually receives inner identity as gift and outcome.

The language here employed now verges on a religious statement of the problem. The insight therapists resemble the latter-day Lutherans and Protestant liberals of the nineteenth century who sharply distinguished between the inner and the outer man, and therefore between an authentic spiritual life and mere external form and ceremony.[29] These Protestants associated a concern for form and ceremony with Catholicism and with the corrupting influence of Roman legalism on Christian faith. External practices signify nothing except as they express interior faith. Without faith and grace all external pieties ring hollow.

The alternative religious tradition values external ritual and piety more highly. The habits of worship and the discipline of prayer and other daily rites help prepare the soul for the eventual vision of God and also help sustain it during those arid stretches when faith seems to have withered. External practices help the soul through its "dark night," absent all vision. Philosophically, such convictions about the moral life trace back to Aristotle, who did not rely too heavily on direct, immediate inspiration, but rather on the prosaic upbuilding of external habits. For this reason, Aristotle did not hesitate to compare ethics—skill in living—with other skills such as athletics and crafts that depend heavily on habits strengthened and sharpened through practice.

While theoreticians tend to see these approaches to religion, ethics, and therapy as opposing types, therapists who work with the physically battered borrow eclectically from both schools. They attempt to offer insight, and they espouse exercise. Such eclectics may be acting wisely. These two schools of therapy may, in fact, contribute to one another. The analogy from the theater suggests as much. How could an Olivier begin with the externals of voice, posture, and gait unless he had some, albeit obscure, insight into the direction in which he had to move? How could a Brando envisage and attain some kind of inner identity with the character he would play unless his own body helped tutor him in the truth and the counterfeit?

Not until recently has Western society and its courts recognized battery within the family as a legitimate interest of the state and cause for compassionate intervention. The government's resources must supplement those of churches and recently emergent mutual support groups in sheltering battered individuals and nurturing beleaguered families, even though it may be too early to assess definitively the relative merits of specific types of treatment. Whether therapists and their charges opt for insight or exercise or some combination of both, they work still by faith rather than by sight. But, in any event, they and their clients have begun to bet their vocation and lives on an "as if," as if the chains will break if one begins to behave and to perceive in a different manner.

THE MOLESTED

THE MOLESTED, like the battered, live in a world of pain, not strictly medical, but which often turns up first in the emergency rooms of hospitals—conspicuously but mutely. The sexual violation or the bruises show, but the victims often do not speak. Since not all victims report the crimes of molestation and incest, one can only guess at their frequency. Some experts estimate that as many as one in four girls in the United States have, at one time or another, suffered sexual abuse.[1] Others put the figure as low as 2 percent. Three different studies of college students (as distinct from more restricted studies of victims treated in clinics) agree enough to suggest that 10 to 19 percent of women students have suffered, as girls, a long-term, abusive, sexual relationship.[2] That percentage does not include single episodes of indecent exposure or fondling.

Mothers routinely warn their sons and daughters to beware of strangers. But, in 75 to 80 percent of sex offenses against children, the child knew and first trusted, or should have had reason to trust, the victimizer.[3] Not an outsider in the alley but an insider in the home or an adult in a trusted role abuses the child. Forty-four percent of abusers in David Finkelhor's study of male and female college students were family members, 22 percent, members of the nuclear family, and 6 percent, fathers or stepfathers.

This chapter will concentrate on abuse by fathers and stepfathers, not because such abuse predominates but because it structurally exposes the abuse of power, intimacy, and trust. This chapter will also concentrate on the abuse of girls. Earlier clinical studies suggested that women suffered abuse as children seven to nine times more often than men, but more comprehensive, nonclinical studies decrease that ratio to two to one. (The boy's experience of abuse is largely but not exclusively homosexual.)

Therapists report that some of the victims manage to do well in spite of the scars. But many do not. Abuse and incest, for example, can eroticize victims and thus distort their perceptions of self and others. They don't know the difference between sexual and nonsexual touch. Thus they themselves proposition inappropriately. The sexual serves as a prism through which they see everything; it limits other areas of their development. The specific nature of the sexual experience will also skew their preferences: some abused girls will, for example, turn on to older men, anal sex, or other unlikely gratifications.

Incest precedes or accompanies a vast array of human troubles, many of which persist long after the abuser, for reasons of fear or discovery, has stopped molesting the victim. A forty-year-old woman still finds it difficult to recount episodes of incest without fearing that she will lose her home. Thirty-eight-year-old Charlotte Vale Allen comes home at night still expecting "The Man with the Knife" to attack her.[4] Incest produces anxiety, depression, flashback terrors, guilt, shame, humiliation, pain, suffering, anger, fear, confusion, and a terrible isolation. It also causes a variety of disturbances in behavior: overeating, anorexia, prostitution (two-thirds to three-fourths of teenage prostitutes have suffered incestuous assault in childhood),[5] other forms of sexual dysfunction, alcoholism, drug abuse (some 40 to 70 percent of adolescent drug addicts are victims of incest), sleep disturbance, runaway and suicidal behavior (75 percent of runaway children are seeking escape from incestuous abuse). In later life, incest victims often suffer from frigidity, sometimes behave promiscuously, sometimes unwittingly encourage incestuous behavior in their own families. In one study, over 75 percent of sex offenders in prison had suffered sexual abuse as children and 80 percent of their wives had suffered sexual abuse as children.

General statistics, however, about the scope and impact of incest do not illustrate the problem as well as specific cases. For example, Dr. Alayne Yates, professor of psychiatry and pediatrics at the University of Arizona, has published the case of two girls who, at four and six years of age, were taken by authorities from their retarded mother and placed in the hands of a foster mother after their natural father had abused and raped them.[6] Their father apparently "did everything" to the two girls and to yet two other children (their three-year-old and six-month-old brothers, whom the father also raped but whom the foster mother had not taken in as charges). According to the foster mother's testimony, the two girls knew nothing about caring for themselves at the toilet, taking a bath, or dressing themselves. They ate dog food. Even after two years in the foster home, the older girl, now eight, has remained sexually active. She will proposition any male, offering and efficiently proceeding to oral sex. She also plays with little girls, but she prefers boys. In her new foster home, she took up with a seventeen-year-old foster son, whom the authorities eventually removed to a detention home and then to the home of the foster mother's sister, while the foster mother tried to bring the little girl's behavior under control.

The woman's strategy?[7] "I punish her when she does wrong things by standing her in a corner for ten minutes. If she stops, I give her a star, and, with ten stars, she gets a nickel." But the foster mother's petty threats and enticements haven't changed the girl's habits. The little girl speaks matter of factly of the powerful draw of sexual pleasure. "It feels me good, so I do it to myself. Everyday. My mom catch me at it. My mom has me stand up with my hands up. I would really like to stop but it feels good."

"Why would you want to stop if it feels so good?"

"Yeah, but you can be put in jail." That threat she reports in a telltale, singsong, tone. Jail sounds abstract. The pleasure is concrete.

"Could you stop for a whole week if I'd give you an ice cream cone?"

"Maybe, but nothing else feels as good as those nasties. I done it in school and on the school bus. I sit way, way back. I like to do it because it feels good. I like doing it with the boys most. Dad did it to my brother's behind. He didn't put it all the way in. It's big. But it didn't hurt me. It feels me good."

The little girl reports another episode: "I sucked on his wiener. He told me to do it. The boy was put in jail."

"How did you feel about it?"

"Happy. But sad because he was put in jail."

"Do you want to get married?"

"Yeah."

"What kind of man do you want to marry? Who do you want to marry?"

"Whatever I get. I like being mother. I got a monkey, and a raggedy. I want to take care of my baby and have my husband take care of the baby when he goes to the doctor."

"Does nasty stuff have anything to do with having babies?"

"No."

"How do they get here?"

"From the mommy."

"How do they come out?"

"I don't know how they get out. I guess they cut it open and sew it back up."

In cases such as this, the foster mother, or adopting parents, can hope, at best, for very little. Ten stars and a nickel do not compete with the turn-on. Nothing feels as good as that. Further, the foster mother's offer of a nickel for ten stars does not compare with the cash the boy in the back of the bus will pay. For the immediate future, at least, the foster mother cannot possibly eliminate or much modify the girl's sexual activity. She can only hope to contain it, or, with the help of responsible adults, to banish it from public settings—from the bus, the school, and the living room—and let the girl masturbate in the privacy of the bedroom. There is no route back to innocence.

In her published comments on her interviews with the little girls, Dr. Yates observes that the eroticized child "may be not only the victim but a participant."[8] Yates characterizes the child as a participant on the grounds that most incest goes unreported and lasts, on the average, three years. "Reluctance to report the incest is due in part to the child's shame, guilt, and fear of reprisal; however, it is also related to the gratification that the incest provides the child."[9] In interpreting the child as a participant, Yates wants to disabuse the reader of a superficial understanding of the child's (and the therapist's) problem. Seduced as well as forced, the eroticized child may consent, cooperate, and seek pleasure, rather than merely submit.

But this view of the child as a compliant, even eager participant does not make her less a victim. In a sense, her cooperation shows how thoroughly the predator has victimized her. Those who forcefully enslave leave open a chance for freedom; those who convince the slave to believe she enjoys slavery have taken her completely, body and soul. The girl's testimony disturbs us because we realize how readily she and, indeed, most children try to accept as normal, internalize, and adapt to the world they have received from their parents no matter how bizarre and destructive it may be. The girl has so conscientiously accepted her training, so eagerly attuned her sense of pleasure and decorum to the picture her father has forced on her, so generously shared her little store of expertise with her peers, that she lets us see, in all innocence, how truly and profoundly and totally he has made her a victim.

When seduced and traduced for the first time at a later age (more usually the victim is eight or nine), the child may accept the father's world less pliantly. She may, in a sense, resist more but she suffers no less. Like the battered spouse, she resembles the victim in the Gothic novel. The lord of the house, whose home, after all, is his castle, rules there and wholly isolates his victim behind thick walls, a broad moat, and a lifted drawbridge. She must do the lord's bidding. He may not entirely control her mind, but he can threaten or hurt her body, and he can dispense a series of rewards and punishments that establish more prisons within the prison.

Often the mother lacks the power to help. She may have already, wittingly or unwittingly, abandoned the child. She may so associate any and all touching with the erotic that she cannot hug her children. Or, in withdrawal from her own past sexual servitude, she may, in effect, throw her daughter off the sled to the father. But the mother's possible rejection or withdrawal does not make the molester a victim. Most fathers and stepfathers, after all—whatever the relations between their wives and daughters—do not seize that opportunity to lure their daughters into what they cloak as "a little game . . . our secret; just the two of us."[10]

The father's opening ploy of the "game" deceives: the playfulness of the setting, the apparent harmlessness of it all. He pretends that playing around will not exploit the deepest springs of vulnerability, power, and want. "It's only a game," such a father says; "our little secret won't shatter the world with which you are already familiar." He thus exploits a gamboling, fuzzy, drowsy innocence. Games, after all, include lots of little secrets, signals, and private jokes between friends.

These disarming comments about the harmlessness of play perpetrate a lie and keep cheating the victim. One victim reported:

"'And you really mean it, this is what all little girls and their daddies do?'

'Didn't I tell you, eh?'

'I know. But if everybody does it, then how come I can't tell?'"[11]

However, when the attacker sensed possible discovery, he harshly stuffed the child under the covers and betrayed his fear of the dynamite he was playing with. Confused, she asked:

"'Why'd you *do* that. You *scared* me!'

'Be quiet!' he hissed. 'You want them to find out what's going on? Christ! . . . . you almost got us caught.'"[12]

The father, fearing discovery, then thickened the walls against the outside world with threats:

"'Don't you tell *anyone* ever!'

'You want me to go to prison?'

'They'd put you away too.'"

Other such molesters warn that if the victim lets the secret out, they will commit suicide. Or they may browbeat their victims by predicting, "Your mother would commit suicide." And, "It will be your fault." If she blurts out the secret, she will not bring a rescuer but intruders who will destroy the family.

After slamming the gates shut against help from the outside world, the father dominates her yet further. With threats and inducements, he weakens her will and freedom. He knows where all the levers are. If she balks at doing what he wants, he takes it out on her and the rest of the family. He treats the girl as the tyrannized wife, a beleaguered peacemaker. He gets angry and lashes out at others but blames her, and she believes him. If she plays his games, he will pay her. The pay locks her in still further, since she now sees herself as consenting and therefore corrupt, cooperating with her corrupt father. Thus, step by step he leads an eight-year-old into playing, at one and the same time, the roles of the self-sacrificing wife and the whore.

Incest violates the child at the deepest possible levels—by bruising not the body but the inner sanctum, the child's very identity. She senses her self not confidently, as loved, but as exploited, eroticized. An identity, still obscure to the self, makes itself felt now, not in the urgency of love but in a "sick, twisty, horrible feeling."[13]

Suffering twists and wrenches the core self out of shape or splits it in two.

> Two quite different girls: one was the sharer of the Secret, who had more money than she knew what to do with, and a strange, almost unpleasant sense of power because of it . . . the One was evil mean, capable of everything bad. The Other was the little girl who played hopscotch and double-Dutch, who romped with Marianna [who] heard screaming voices, couldn't eat, couldn't concentrate, felt scared and on edge all the time, and dreamed non-stop of a nice future, of having a loving family, of being left alone . . . [she] . . . was the me the world at large saw out on her best behavior, in the hope that someone would see and value her.[14]

Another describes the distortion and split a little less melodramatically but no less poignantly.

> She enjoyed her father's caresses . . . yet she felt guilty about the incest. She felt competitive with her mother and yet unable to communicate with her. She became promiscuous, yet mistrusted men. She was enraged at her father's betrayal of her trust and violation of her physical integrity, and at her mother's failure to protect her.[15]

In a study of "Long Term Effects of Childhood Incest on Adult Women,"[16] Dennis L. Bull notes the conflicting responses of clinging dependency and emotional distancing, opposites, to be sure, and yet they often appear at the same time in the same woman. Although she has broken from the original molester, she still seeks out substitute authority figures and yet dissociates from intimacy. She inwardly distances herself by repeating the child's ploy of the "possum defense."[17] The possum child lies preternaturally still during the abuse, pretending to sleep or, alternatively, pretending to leave her body "and coldly watch from a corner of the room or fade into the wall and watch what was happening. . . ."[18]

Eventually the incest victim may try to insulate herself from the rape through alcohol, drug abuse, fantasies, suicide, or compulsive eating and/or fasting. Already walled off from the outside world during the abuse, the incest victim now attempts to build an inner wall between herself and what her attacker did to her. If incest, in effect, breaks a taboo, if it breaks down the primordial wall between father and daughter, brother and sister, uncle and niece, stepfather and stepdaughter, then the various desperate strategies of distancing erect still other walls to hide the broken wall.

The "possum effect" and the strategy of distancing lead to more than the obviously disturbed efforts to drink, drug, or eat one's way into oblivion. Playing possum extends throughout the victim's life. What we sometimes understatedly call a lack of self-confidence shows up in the person who solves his or her problems through stillness, on the assumption that anything that moves draws bullets. The moving target attracts the eye. The self that stirs is instantly vulnerable. If it moves, it must prepare to duck, or collaborate, or, if not collaborate, resist. The possum self finds that the attacker has stolen or destroyed the appetite, the resource, the ability, the self-confidence to do any of these.

SECRECY

The literature on incest, including this essay, emphasizes secrecy. Different members of the family, for varying reasons, build a thick wall of silence and lies between the family and others. The father, often conservative and authoritarian, fortifies the line against others partly out of resentment and fear. He alone commands the family. But, his fear-driven defensiveness does not entirely explain his line-drawing. His incest itself often springs from a kind of family tribalism, a perverted righteousness. He would consider philandering outside of the family immoral. Ordinary adultery would betray the family to an outsider. Seducing his daughter keeps fornication, as it were, in the family. The collusive mother reinforces the family secret partly out of her shame, partly out of her fear of destroying the family, and perhaps partly out of her collaboration in the incest. The victim's intense feelings of shame, fear, and guilt also make it well-nigh impossible for her to reveal the secret to others. When she does blurt out the secret, she often will deny her disclosure with a retraction, desperately trying to recant what she has decanted.

But Dr. Yates's interviews with the six- and eight-year-old girls reveal that the degree and kind of secrecy varies, depending on the child's age and maturity. Their youth and early training in incest led these girls to speak openly and matter of factly of the "nasties." Indeed, their candid talk and behavior disturbed others on the bus, in school, and at home, with the obliviousness of the corrupted innocent. They remind us that the preschool child accepts the world as it comes to her from the hands of her parents. Since her parents define the normal, she cannot think of them as abnormal. Her parents can do nothing that requires hiding. Little children, of course, play games and keep secrets. But they understand a game as "special" rather than lethal. They do not yet understand that the molester and the society at large put the game of incest into the category not of the special but of the abnormal and the forbidden.

The secret changes from an invitational to a forbidden game. As the child grows and consorts with others at school she begins to realize, as did Charlotte Vale Allen, that things differ in other families. She now discovers herself submitting to a game that stimulates shame, perhaps compassion, and guilt. As she approaches puberty and wants to see and be with boys, the father jealously constrains her, and powerful currents of anger, resentment, abiding grief and grievance surge through her. She sees her abuser, the enforcer of the secret, as her jailor. But breaking out of jail doesn't free her. She carries with her emotion and training that tragically dispose her to repeat in her own life choices that her abuser originally forced on her as fate. Sandra Butler reports of one such, "she said she felt like he had her in a prison and wouldn't let her out." She had no boy friends, no life outside the house. And yet, later, when "on her own," she substituted an abusive, authoritarian pimp for the abusive, authoritarian incestuous father.[19]

GUILT

Guilt and shame mount guard as sentinels to keep the secret secure. The victim's guilt reflects snarled relations to others; shame betrays her lowered self-esteem. Guilt weighs doubly on the child, both forcing her to keep the secret from the outside world and driving her to comply further with her father's wishes. The father threatens with and blames her for the horrific consequences of disclosure and she comes to believe that only further compliance will save the family. If she blurts out the secret, she will send Daddy to jail, upset Mother, and drive Mommy to suicide. She will break up the family; and the authorities will scatter brothers and sisters to foster homes. Moreover, she feels guilt not only about those evils which she believes she will bring down on the family but also because her abuser has convinced her that she provoked the relationship in the first instance and cannot abandon what she has begun.

Molesters are masters in using passive language to describe their actions. "Then it happened" (as though "it" were a downdraft of air that swept him along impersonally like a newspaper tumbling in the gutter). Or, "the hand was touching her clitoris" (as though the hand connected only incidentally with his own person). Or, "her breast was put in my mouth" (as though the little girl mounted a stepladder to accost her six-foot father). Or, "she didn't do anything to stop it," as though she, not he, bore responsibility. The abuser uses this passive language, threats, and manipulations to make her feel responsible for initiative in the enterprise, a not too difficult maneuver since, as Dr. Yates observes, sex does turn her on.

Finally, the girl feels guilt because she has often, in fact, supplanted her mother as sexual partner. She also has accepted disproportionately large maternal responsibilities for her siblings (sometimes assuming, wrongly, that by acceding to her abuser's demands she will protect her sisters and brothers from similar demands). The girl, after all, has won the Electra contest. Thus, if she blurts out the family secret and destroys the family, she does not do so simply as a daughter who herself someday must leave the family in her own right, but as the mother who has in a sense destroyed her own—a terrible load of guilt to bear. No wonder such a victim, Charlotte Vale Allen, suffers recurrent nightmares of an avenging figure come to punish her. Incest corrupts not by enforcing physical powerlessness but by imposing sexual power on the child prematurely.

The results in many cases seem to confirm the child's own feeling of guilt. The thirteen-year-old girl with a bladder infection and venereal disease eventually confesses that "Daddy did it to me." The doctor examines her a second time, this time asking all sorts of questions about Daddy. Medical authorities turn her over to the precinct station where the police take up the case. But, under various pressures, she recants her story and he goes free. Until recent years, authorities sent the girl to juvenile hall, where she waited to be placed in an institution or a foster home. Unavoidably, she felt that "being taken out of her home was punishment for what she did. Her guilt is sealed in silence and withdrawal."[20] More usually today, the successfully prosecuted offender is sent away. Either way, the family suffers hardship. If she had kept quiet, she believes, the family would not have undergone that stress.

SHAME

However victimized, the abused child cannot console herself by thinking of herself solely as a victim. Though forced to serve her father, she cannot wholly excuse herself. In fact, she loathes herself. He has managed to pollute her core. She feels "so dirty, God so dirty. I'm dirty, horribly dirty."[21] Modern liberal culture associates guilt and shame with personal responsibility. It does not illumine the polluting touch that stains an unconsenting or resisting child.

In his study of alcoholics, Ernest Kurtz contrasts the two spiritual states of guilt and shame. "Guilt reveals itself in self-reproaches that run: How could I have *done that*; what an injurious *thing* to have done; how could I hurt *so-and-so*; what a moral lapse that *act* was! Simultaneously, however, shame induces self-reproaches with a very different emphasis: how could *I* have done that; what an *idiot* I am; what a *fool*; how awful and worthless *I am*."[22]

In a culture of guilt one condemns lies because they wrong and harm others. In a culture of shame one condemns lies because they diminish the liar. But shame does not spring exclusively from self-condemnation. Certainly our shabby treatment of others can provoke our own sense of self-diminution. This feeling strengthens when others learn what we have done, or, more precisely, as we learn that they know. Our shabby deeds suddenly expose us to view; others see what we have done and reprove us. Thus, our shameful sense that we do not enjoy or deserve the esteem of others further lowers our already lowered self-esteem.

People in a shame-sensitive culture want honors; they prize the approval of others. They seek to prove their mettle and worth. A challenge proves one true or false, worthy or spurious. During a "moment of truth," a person shows his stuff, displays his or her quality. Such a moment reveals not abstract truth, but the truth the early Greeks called *Aliethiea*, stepping forth into the open, out of hiding. (The Greek epic *Aliethiea* required two participants—the warrior to perform the deed and the poet to celebrate it. The two let a hero step forth and show his quality.) Correspondingly, an honorable person acts openly and straightforwardly, shows openly what, in fact, deserves approbation. Oppositely, the person who feels shame must hide the dreadful exposed lack he has shown, his failure as a man. He knows that he has fallen short and the community finds him wanting. It esteems him not and he loses self-esteem.

In ordinary life, shame impels us to hide what we ought to hide. The site of shame is the exposed backside (spanking punishes by shaming). When something we normally take pride in behaves shamefully, we reflexively seek to hide it from view. The victim of incest suffers massive shame: incest has exposed not only her body but her entire family and reduced it to a bare bottom. She can no longer feel pride in her family openly and straightforwardly; pride persists only defensively in the form of keeping secret what she dare not expose to view. Thus shame resembles a tropical forest; it throws its damp shade everywhere, and secrecy luxuriates beneath it.

The little girl who tells all and brings everything into the open lives beyond pride or shame. Not that she has placed herself there; her victimizer must take the credit for that. But she reminds us that "shame" and "shameless" do not oppose one another as do "guilt" and "guiltless." While "guiltless" means "without guilt," "shameless" does not mean to be without reason for shame. Rather, we call a person "shame-less" who seems to have lost, or not to have acquired, the ability to feel shame. "Shameless" suggests a person disconnected from the human, a moral vacuum, as it were, who cannot feel a decent respect for the opinion of humankind.

The person who cannot feel shame reminds one of the Grimms' fairy tale about the little boy who could not shudder.[23] His defective sensibility led him to behave inappropriately—he played, for example, with a corpse and his parents eventually banished him. He had, in effect, crossed the border into the nonhuman. Similarly, the shameless person seems to have crossed the border beyond human community. He blurts out what we all want concealed or, at least, revealed only with reticence, and therewith he reveals his inability, as it were, to blush, a defect in humanity that resembles the inability to shudder.[24] The prophet Cassandra similarly disturbs because she prophesies what we must hide; she sees, like the child, the Emperor's nakedness and speaks out, without the constraints that ordinarily mark and bind the human.

Reports from foster parents and adopting parents indicate that the eroticized child, through no fault of her own, does not fit smoothly into a new family unit. Like the family in the Grimms' fairy tale, the foster and adopting parents soon feel compelled to send such a child on her way. She bounces from home to home or from institution to institution. Such a movement from affectless home to alien family quickly reconfirms her plight as a renegade without the capacity to connect or to feel either common shame or trust.

INCEST AS A *TABU*

Some relativists would argue that the experience of shame has no objective cause. They attribute shame to the breach of a socially established, and therefore essentially arbitrary, *tabu*. Theoretically, then, one might relieve the psychological destruction of incest simply by lifting the *tabu*. Eliminate the border and the damages from border-crossing disappear.

This essay has generally argued exactly the reverse: the *tabu* does not create the danger; it protects the child and the entire family from danger and devastation. The *tabu* is not a social absurdity; it makes moral sense.

Arguments for the *tabu* against incest usually begin with biology and genetics.[25] Inbreeding weakens and degenerates a gene pool. Deleterious genes at length vitiate the descendants of incestuous kinship groups. However, the long-range consequence of oft-repeated inbreeding would not of itself rule out the occasional exception. Nor would it explain the *tabu* against incest in traditional societies that lacked the sophistication of modern genetics and yet forbade the practice.

A second, social argument treats the *tabu* as a protection against already powerful centripetal tendencies in the family. Incest reinforces those inward-moving tendencies that already ripple through displays of affection in family life: the infant who locks his eyes with his mother in mirthful dance; the girl who takes pride and pleasure in the attractiveness of her father and brother; children who bask in the knowledge that their parents find them, at least occasionally, entrancing. If members of the family let their relatively innocent, open, and diffuse feelings change over and close down into sexual love, then the family, already a walled community, ends up a windowless monad.

Marriage outside the family thus carries and spreads tendrils from the family into a wider community. It keeps the family open to the strange and the stranger. The term *hetero*sexual love—love of the strange self, the stranger to oneself but also to one's family—reminds one that love and life attract the stranger. The opening to the strange ventilates and strengthens both families and the community at large.

The strongest justification for the *tabu* against incest rests upon the parents' duty to protect and foster the being and well-being of their children in the midst of a necessary dependency that can become nearly lethal. Human offspring depend upon their parents more intensively and extensively than do the offspring of any other species. Parenting always runs close to the border of failure by creating in the child a permanent and crippling dependency. When parents, however, seduce their children, they geometrically compound the original dependency with a second, sexual dependency. This double dependency grievously hinders children in becoming adults in their own right and turn. It imposes upon the child a paralyzing vulnerability, an immobilizing shame, a terrible confusion in perception of the parental role and the child's own.

Even at best, sexual love entails vulnerability, and, as such, always borders on shame. In sexual love, the hungering, needy self must expose itself. Sexual desires unveil; one entrusts oneself into the hands of another. One sees the other's weakness and need. Thus, however imperiously the parent may behave in the sexual relationship, the child sees the parent as pathetic, wanting, and needing. Whether the child responds or not, the parent deprives her of her childhood by effacing himself as a powerful protector and handing her instead a weak and needing lover. The child, not yet an adult, needs her protected childhood in order to grow. She needs a parent who will support her own flourishing—a parent who will point her toward that day when she will have grown strong enough to survive the vulnerability of love.

BETRAYAL AND THE BETRAYERS

The victim experiences betrayals. First and foremost, the abuser has betrayed her—whether as father, stepfather, mother's boyfriend, older brother, or yet another authority figure whom she would, under ordinary circumstances, trust. (Too often in this essay, I have referred to the father and not, as I should, to the father figure. Stepfathers commit incest five times more often than fathers. Live-in boyfriends are also an exceptionally high risk.) The abuser violates the child's right to respect and treatment as a child, to protection from the world, and to counsel in interpreting its ambiguities. Instead, he throws her into a whirlpool of feelings and experiences that she cannot swim away from. Or he seductively offers himself as a lifeline, only to turn into a chain that drags her into the vortex of the whirlpool. The apparent deliverer is himself the enemy into whose hands she is delivered.

At least two differing types of men commit incest: the Don Juan and the Patriarch. The inveterate womanizer takes his opportunities wherever he finds them. The wife usually knows he womanizes, but does not know that he fails to respect the home as off-limits. He may view taking his daughter or stepdaughter as nothing more than "breaking her in," his seignorial privilege. While this type of molester respects no boundaries, the second (the Patriarch, whom we have already described) perversely respects his own territorial boundaries and keeps assiduously within them. He would not think of fornicating outside the clan. He abhors and forbids extrafamilial sex. This second type often goes regularly to church and wields conservative authority within the family.

The perpetrator will usually deny the abuse, by calling the girl a liar, or deny his guilt, either by calling the girl the aggressor or by lapsing, as mentioned earlier, into the passive voice or the impersonal mode.

Although the victimizer may wield in the house total power over the child, in the outside world, the experts report, he has often failed at work or found rejection in one setting or another. Like his victim, he also suffers from low self-esteem. When caught and imprisoned, he discovers that other prisoners condemn him: "the other prisoners don't want anything to do with me. They treat me like I'm the lowest of the low."[26]

The mother has also betrayed her child, by failing to protect her daughter from the predator, by withdrawing from the home or from acknowledging the incest, thus abandoning the child, or, in some cases, by actively collaborating in the abuse. Girls who live without their mothers suffer abuse three times as often as those whose mothers live in the house. However, even when present, some mothers are often absent: either frequently ill, emotionally distant, often unaware, subordinate to the husband, or disbelieving. In 6 percent of the cases, she collaborates with the father. The mother, who ordinarily should irradiate a home with a sense of protected well-being, now, through her absence, ionizes empty space for the sexually abused child with a sense of danger.

Eighty percent of the mothers of incest victims themselves suffered sexual abuse as children.[27] The sexually molested woman sometimes withdraws as a wife, clearing the father's way to the daughter. Butler found that mothers who had endured incest themselves sometimes also distanced themselves from their children; "all touching was so weighted with painful memories that they were unable to feel a closeness with and freedom to touch their own children."[28] This double withdrawal transfers wifely and maternal responsibilities to the daughter. When the mother finds out about the incest, she often blames the daughter or sticks by the husband as the better of two bad deals. Her refusal to participate in the effort to rehabilitate can increase the daughter's (and her own) sense of guilt.

The person in whom the child eventually confides may betray the victim a third time. Guilt-stricken, ashamed, and fearful, she finds it hard enough to reveal her plight. But then the person to whom she reports her troubles may not take her seriously. After all, she has called an intimate or trusted friend of the family a predator. The confused girl may suffer from a lack of credibility, especially since she may blurt out her difficulty only after she has already created a record of erratic and rebellious behavior. Her interlocutor may easily dismiss her and, in not a few cases, the person in whom she confides may think of her as soiled goods and treat her confidence as an invitation to try predation on his own.

In addition to these personal betrayals, the girl may feel that her own body has betrayed her. It may have responded to the stimulus and provoked her to participate and consent. One victim reports, "My body just betrayed me." I felt "double-crossed by my own body."[29]

And why not yield? In effect, the very meaning of the family has collapsed for the child. The modern family, as Christopher Lasch has observed, functions less as a working unit within the larger world than as a haven and respite from it. But for the abused or battered child that haven has become heartbreak hill, the place where adults who have restrained their combative and predatory instincts elsewhere now give them free play. The father who may be too timid to sweet-talk a grown woman into an erotic agenda can manipulate, intimidate, and trick a child.

THERAPY

The moral and theological reasons for helping the victims of battering and incest need no elaboration: the government and all other institutions and persons able to help must protect and assist the abused. The theological tradition states this imperative with the full force of the voice of God. God identifies himself with the cause of the voiceless and the powerless. That declaration and the moral imperatives that follow from it reverberate through the prophets of Israel and the teachings of Jesus.

The reasons for helping batterers and molesters are less obvious. The glowering face of attorney Joel Steinberg, on trial during the winter of 1988–89 for regularly beating and then finally and fatally abandoning his adopted daughter, Lisa, aroused moral indignation throughout the nation. Can a society move beyond abhorring the crime and punishing the criminal? Can it justify reaching out to the abuser? Or does a single step in that direction betray the innocent and the powerless?

The moral arguments for helping the abuser divide into the instrumental and the independent. Instrumentally, one can argue that, short of jailing the abuser and throwing away the key, one can protect potential future victims only by rehabilitating the abuser. Further, past victims may also profit from his rehabilitation. Clearly, the battered or molested member of the family suffers not only the pain of physical injury but also the violation of a personal relation. The abuser's rehabilitation can aid in restoring that relationship. His recovery can thereby help close a painful chapter in his victim's life, even though no further contacts occur between them. While the victim's recovery does not altogether depend upon the redemption of the abuser, his rehabilitation can help.

Independently, the moral reason for offering help to the victimizer, beyond its benefits for the victim, rests on the Kantian dictum that one must always respect persons. Kant rightfully argued that such respect does not require that one must never use persons as means to other ends, but rather that one must never use them as means *only*. One owes respect and help to all persons as ends in themselves, however much they may have injured others and abased themselves.

The theological warrant in the Christian tradition for helping the batterer and the molester similarly takes two forms. First and instrumentally, full protection and redemption of the abused and powerless, whose cause God makes his own (Matthew 24:31–46), require the rehabilitation of those predators with whom their lives, for better or for worse, intertwine. Second and independently, the Christian tradition identifies God, under the form of his servant and son, with even the despised and the rejected, those from whom men hide their faces and esteem them not, and "he makes intercession for the transgressors" (Isaiah 53:12). The authors of the gospels see Jesus' calling within the suffering servant passages of Isaiah, "He took our infirmities and bore our diseases" (Matthew 8:17). These passages hardly justify minimizing the crimes or sentimentalizing the mindset that produced them. On the contrary, God's powerful love, which reaches out toward all creatures, judges the petty tyrannies, the sad exploitations, and the mawkish self-pity that figure in beating and molesting. At the same time, however, that love demands that others of his creatures not rule out of the human race those whom God himself has not chosen to place beyond the pale.

These moral and religious considerations justify therapy and argue further for forms of therapy that do not simply compound the problems of the principals in abuse. The girl, for example, can suffer yet a further betrayal when she finally gets through to the authorities, and they take over. Officials can run away with the case, sending the father to prison, shipping her to a foster home, and breaking up the family. The trauma calls for therapy, but therapy itself imposes a trauma. While the victim needs to learn how to transfer responsibility for what has happened to the predator, the molester and his silent partner (if the mother has colluded) must learn how to accept it. The molester often listens to professionals who offer contrary advice. Lawyers tell him to respond tactically and defensively: admit only what you must and no more. It will go badly for you. The more you admit, the longer the jail sentence and the smaller the chances of enrolling in a substitute or supplementary treatment program. Don't enroll in a treatment program too soon: you may appear to admit guilt. Therapists, on the other hand, emphasize the importance of honest admission in a successful recovery. Legal strategy encourages dodgy behavior; but effective treatment requires the molester to admit and reckon with the full enormity of his incest.

If the girl does not retract her charges (in fact, she often does: 80 percent of the cases are not prosecuted) and if the court sustains them, the molester finally serves a jail sentence and/or, in some states, participates in mandated treatment. In Arizona, for example, the courts sentence the convicted molester to up to a year in jail, but often in a work-release program. He lives in jail, but can work to support his family. If he enrolls successfully in a treatment program, the court will award him released time for therapy. The treatment program thus often runs concurrent with his jail sentence and extends through another three to seven years during probation.

Treatment programs reduce recidivism greatly, but the admissions committees for some such programs screen out in advance the probable recidivists. The least promising candidates include those men who have molested more than one child (whether in the home or elsewhere), those who use force or violence (the abuser usually tries coercively to seduce rather than overtly to force), or those addicted to alcohol or drugs. One should not infer from the low figures on recidivism that the programs rehabilitate the molester totally. The programs may modify his behavior without, however, eliminating his main problems.

Insight therapists in the field generally concede that therapists must also use behavior modification programs. The molester clearly needs to modify his behavior, with or without understanding his deeper problems. And incest victims, as well, urgently need to behave differently, whether they remain in their own home or move to a foster home. The foster family cannot incorporate the child unless she changes her behavior. The eroticized or distrustful child can create havoc in family life. Thus foster parents will avoid accepting the victims of incest in the first place or, discovering the problem, will return the already accepted child to other custody. Thus children bounce from foster home to foster home; these rejections confirm their sense that those near to them will betray or abandon them. Children come to distrust, and for good empirical reasons, any and all human ties. Their would-be rescuers only confirm the lesson which the incestuous molester taught them first: beneath all appearances, the human heart is cold.

The need to modify or control the child's behavior to help her live successfully in a new family only pushes the responsibility for training back one step onto the adopting parents or foster parents. They will need to help the child change bad habits, widen pleasures, and create some habits lacking before—an undertaking for which earlier experience may not have equipped them. Who can train the trainers? The lack of training programs for foster and adopting parents deeply weakens current therapeutic programs. A Minneapolis program, among a few others, trains the foster family to handle the victims of incest. Reports from Texas and elsewhere[30] suggest that adoptive parents resent current state practices that persuade them to take a child without informing them either of the incest or of the behavioral problems that sometimes (not always) follow, and without providing the parents special training and supports. Embittered parents feel that the state has first conned and then abandoned them. Such emotional turbulence only repeats and strengthens afresh the child's perception of abandonment.

Behavior modification (in the setting of group therapy) can help the victim, but alone it will not suffice. Some group work merely deteriorates into a collective venting of anger. That approach alone does not solve the specific problem the victims face, since they have felt not only anger but also love, erotic love. Ultimately, the badly abused child needs professional therapy. The two young girls in the case presented by Dr. Yates with which we began have obviously normalized their little store of squalid experience and so matter of factly assimilated it and generously shared it that one cannot imagine successfully restructuring their lives without long-term therapy. They need to restructure their relationships, most particularly, but not only, with men. Such girls need, in Dr. Yates's judgment, a male therapist. But very few male therapists treat victims of incest (partly because the women's movement has claimed incest as its cause, but only partly for that reason). Most male therapists in the field do social work, not psychiatry, and those few male social workers have tended to treat the adult offender, not the victim. Dr. Yates observes wryly that working with the sexually abused is high-risk work for a male. It is fraught with danger. The male therapist faces all the problems of seduction and counter-seduction. The girl may get angry and accuse the man of inappropriate behavior. Still, the restructuring of her relationship to the male presents her greatest problem.

The potential for chaos in any case of incest boggles the imagination. A case includes a variety of primary players (father, mother, victim, siblings, stepfather, uncle, teacher, or mother's boyfriend), a medley of available therapies (behavior modification, psychoanalysis, gestalt therapy, transactional analysis, humanistic psychology, and crisis intervention), and a host of interested agencies and their staffs (medical staff and emergency room personnel, the courts, probation officers, lawyers, social workers, mental health workers, placement agencies, volunteers, and self-help groups such as Parents Anonymous and Parents United). The complexity of the problem and the variety of players and resources require a coordinated community effort. Otherwise the victims, already betrayed and battered, are bounced back and forth between competing institutions, neglected, and/or, in the worst cases, institutionalized.

In response to the need for coordinated effort, the city of Santa Clara, California has mapped out a Comprehensive Child Sexual Abuse Treatment Program.[31] It recognizes and mobilizes three components in sustained and effective therapy: professional treatment, volunteer help, and mutual support groups. While recognizing that the modes of therapy perforce must vary with the case, the program carefully orders the sequence of kinds of treatment and their appropriate targets. For example, conjoint family therapy is "inappropriate for families in the early throes of the crisis."[32] Normally, but not invariably, treatment occurs in the following order: (1) individual counseling, particularly for the child, mother, and father; (2) mother-daughter counseling; (3) marital counseling (crucial if the family wishes to reunite); (4) father-daughter counseling; (5) family counseling; and (6) group counseling.[33] Other family therapists argue that family treatment should begin as soon as possible: to avoid recanting; to communicate apologies; and to signal that the family and its members can work through the ordeal, thereby reducing the likelihood that the victim will bear a load of shame and guilt should the family eventually break up as a unit.

Conventionally, the recidivist rate tests the success of any such program. Normally, the rate of recidivism for this particular crime is 2 percent. The Santa Clara rate reduced the rate to 0.6 percent. But, even more impressive, the number of clients coming forward has increased 40 percent per year over a five-year period. The very existence of the program has helped break the thrall of incest, which depended partly on the family's fear of the consequences that follow from confession or discovery. Thus even if the recidivist rate had not improved, the program would have dramatically increased the number of offenders whose behavior has eventually changed.

Still more important, the program has in most cases successfully restored the girl to her mother and home. The girls spend a median time of 90 days out of the home, and 92 percent can be expected to return to their homes. Given the numbing effects of moving from foster home to foster home, this result particularly encourages optimism. Self-abusive behavior such as drinking, abusing drugs, sexual promiscuity, and running away, and symptoms such as bedwetting, nail-biting, and fainting have declined. Finally, the parents themselves have seen striking improvement in their lives individually and, in many cases, as a couple.

One would not want to suggest that this Santa Clara program should supply the template for all therapeutic efforts to help families mired in incest. But some such comprehensive effort may answer, at least partly, the threat which contemporary efforts to heal so often pose. Incest today occurs largely in a fragmented (as distinct from its earlier setting in a coherent, traditional) society. Inevitably, a fragmented society heightens the isolation which the predator, the victim, and the collaborator feel. The nuclear family, even at its best, often serves as the embattled fortress of which Christopher Lasch complained. At its worst, in cases of incest the family provides thick walls and a moat that conceal the unspeakable. When, moreover, the society responds fragmentarily, its own efforts to liberate only compound the original sense of isolation. The society merely alienates the child and sets her adrift as it moves her from jail to foster home to institution. The Santa Clara program and others like it seek to lessen the additional suffering that institutional fragmentation imposes.

Under the best of circumstances, the very effort to heal the victims of battering and incest imposes its own coefficient of suffering. At best, the molested and battered can look upon rescue and salvation apprehensively and ambivalently. The future hardly rushes toward them, inspiring instant trust and hope. Children can least afford to suffer gratuitously at the hands of their would-be rescuers. Even at their best, therapists and caregivers deprive children of the world they know. They had better not work at cross purposes or without the patience to sustain or the wisdom to guide.

This pain of recovery forces a qualification in the basic pattern adopted for this book—death, perilous passage, and rebirth. The pattern oversimplifies. Sequentially understood, it misleadingly restricts the ordeal of death to the original trauma. We have already conceded that this pattern does not tidily apply to the burn victim. The rigors of treatment also impose upon the victim a battering akin to death.

Similarly, the threat of death does not confront the victim of battering or molestation in the original catastrophe alone. Rehabilitation also menaces and confronts the victim as a death. The plight of the two little girls interviewed by Dr. Yates, albeit bizarre, illustrates the more general problem many other children face. However much their parents abuse them, children, at one level, humbly adjust. They innocently believe that their parents give them the normal world, the real world. They behave like the Spanish Civil War prisoners whom Andre Malraux described in *Man's Hope*, who obediently dug their own graves and then arranged themselves in front of them so that their bodies would fall conveniently into place after their executioners had shot them. Malraux says that these prisoners reminded him of a group of people arranging themselves, at the photographer's request, for a photograph. Thus the terrifying diminishes to the quotidian. Children similarly manage to assimilate what parents hand them, however lethal. But this very assimilation means that later rescue and renewal confront them as destructive. Rescue terrifies, because it does not appear to enrich them or to add to the world they know; it changes and destroys. In its own way, the new world confronts them as a deprivation.

Moreover, after the new life appears to have established itself, the experience of death persists. We have already seen that the parents of the retarded child must endure not only the burial of the dream child when they first discover their child's retardation, but recurrently they will relive that loss as their child reaches specific ages unable to participate fully in the traditional milestones of the normal. However much the mother feels she has anticipated the child's future impairment, her anticipation proves abstract. She will have to bury the dream child all over again, as she discovers specifically that her child will not take music lessons, go off to the conventional camp, learn to drive the car, or graduate from high school. The family must accept anew the different life and identity which, in fact, the child brings.

Similarly, the battered and the molested may repeatedly face the task of setting to rest the past. Even though free from their abusers' immediate control and their new lives begun, they will face, in later times and with other partners, the temptation to fall into old patterns and repeat "unfinished business."[34] The new identity, the reconstructed life, so solid and palpable for some stretches of time, seems dangerously at risk at other times. The victims will face in varying forms and afresh the task of renewal.

THE AGED
Their Virtues and Vices

Two RECOLLECTIONS set the agenda for this chapter. In the first instance, the duty once fell to my wife and me to help an aged woman, a retired librarian, move out of her two-room apartment to a home for the elderly in a nearby town. We barely knew her, except for the coincidence that we had moved to Bloomington, Indiana from the very same city in New England. Clearly her tendency to save and store had run amuck. Newspapers, books, bundles of pencils, papers, rubber bands, string, and every piece of mail that had ever slid through her letter slot filled the apartment from wall to wall, leaving only the most crooked of paths through three- and four-foot hedges of yellowing newspapers. My wife removed the debris and cleaned the apartment, while I readily took on what I thought would be the easier task of driving the woman and her winnowed possessions to the retirement home. My errand had seemed easier because the state of her apartment suggested a woman too senile and oblivious to give me much trouble. But, as we approached the home, which she had seen only once before, she began to tremble uncontrollably. Her shaking reminded me of my English setter, shivering as I left her at the veterinary hospital.

In the second instance, a 78-year-old, heavyset, ebullient woman took care of our four children while my wife and I taught at Smith College. I appreciated her instrumentally. She was very good with the children. But my wife saw more. She also saw in Auntie Holden a model for conduct in her own old age.

These incidents emphasize the two sides to moral reflection about the elderly. Such reflection should include not only the question of our personal and institutional responsibility to them, but also consideration of their moral contributions to others, partly instrumental and partly exemplary.

Accordingly, this chapter falls into two parts. It covers first our moral attitudes toward the elderly and our responsibilities for their care —what Scripture summarizes under the commandment to honor your father and mother. Then it turns to the moral responsibilities of the elderly—what Scripture summarizes under the *Haustafeln*, the table of duties of various members of the human family, in the letter to the Ephesians. The two parts of the chapter connect. Our attitudes toward the elderly and our basic patterns for their care create those specific ordeals with which they must cope and in the midst of which, for better or for worse, their virtues must flourish.

OUR ATTITUDES TOWARD
THE ELDERLY

The British social commentator Ronald Blythe has attributed our increasing neglect of the elderly to their growing numbers.[1] Until recently an older man or woman did not need to succeed to secure honor and respect. Old age itself was a rarity, and, therefore, a kind of success, a performance worthy of honor. Now, however, becoming old is commonplace. The vast majority of Americans and Western Europeans live seven decades; projections suggest eighty-five or so as the natural lifespan; and scientists campaign for funds to develop technologies that will extend life beyond eighty-five. This greying of America and the developed countries may make it harder to keep the filial commandment.

In America, however, neglect of the elderly springs from many causes other than their increased numbers. An attitude of neglect and disrespect particularly tempts an immigrant, perpetually migrant, pragmatic, secular, and proudly independent people. An immigrant country distances itself from forebears. Coming to America entailed a kind of abandonment of the aged. It meant leaving the old country, the land of one's forebears, for a strange land, often without the comfort of one's mother tongue—all for the sake of the young. Immigrants made an extraordinary sacrifice and placed an equally extraordinary pressure on their sons and daughters. In the chapter on the retarded we explored the distortions that this orientation to youth and their achievements imposes on the young. In this chapter we need to acknowledge the negative impacts this obsession with the young places on the elderly. Specifically, the American compulsion to surpass one's parents meant in turn that an immigrant people became a perpetually migrant people. Children left home for college—their first step into the middle class—in quest of better jobs and homes than their parents had, and eventually spilled out of the cities into the suburbs and across the land, hoping to improve their lot, and left their elders behind or saw them off to those territorial nursing homes, Florida and Arizona.

Americans, further, are a pragmatic and a functional people. They tend to identify themselves and others with their doing rather than their being. When retirement strips them of their work, people often forfeit their identity. They lose their self-respect and therefore their hold on the respect of others. The aged thus slip to the margins of consciousness for the ruling generation. America ranks as one of the most secular of countries—not in the modern meaning of secular as irreligious but in its original characterization of a culture that orients to the *current* generation, the generation that holds power and exercises authority. A consumerist society is secular in the sense that it orients with a vengeance to the current generation. It squanders the resources of generations to come and it distances itself from the heritage of generations past all for the sake of the generation now in charge.

But describing the neglect to which secularism leads does not tell the whole story. To the degree that the aged grow in numbers they increasingly threaten the generation in charge. This threat results from their increasing political strength. The elderly have become a power bloc; they have already influenced legislation and court decisions; they have reacquired the right to work beyond age sixty-five and therefore their identity through doing; and they have protected (through Medicare, Medicaid, and cost-of-living adjustments in Social Security payments) their identity through their holdings. Rumblings have already been heard about the great burden of indexed increases in Social Security payments. We may be moving rapidly out of the age of some neglect into an age of resentment and hostility toward the elderly.

That hostility, moreover, may go much deeper than resentment toward their political power. As Blythe has argued, we are dealing with something new in the world, a vanguard horde of the elderly that may increase still further with the development of life-extending technologies. We do not yet know what threats, psychological and otherwise, this population shift will pose for middle-aged adults who are not used to having their elders around for long. At one end, the middle-aged have lengthening responsibilities for dependent youths (adolescence seems to go on forever). And, at the other end, they worry about those who linger indeterminately in their dotage. Middle-aged adults are chiefly responsible for order and provision. Psychologically, they become embattled fortresses—besieged by the young and the old who seem to indulge in endless transition and dependency.

But still deeper than the external burden and threat the aged pose to their adult children lies an internal threat. They remind the middle-aged of their own imminent destiny. The middle aged

frequently find themselves timidly yet compulsively, like tonguing a tooth nerve—measuring their assets against those of youth to see what they have left, and against those of old age to see what has to go. It is often a great deal in both cases. There can be then a spiritual and physical drawing-back from the old, as if they possessed some centrifugal force to drag the no longer young into their slipstream of decay.[2]

The middle-aged fear not only physical decay, the loss of beauty, and the failure of vitality, but humiliating dependency. Americans have traditionally prided themselves as an independent people, beholden to none for political institutions, economic resources, and personal choices. The dark side of this aspiration to self-reliance is an abhorrence of dependency. To depend upon others makes us uneasy; it humiliates us. Philip Slater once observed that Puerto Ricans stranded in New England for the winter found more than the climate cold. The Yankee traditions of independence shut them off from the spontaneous help of others. They missed this feature of their homeland—where to depend on others did not automatically cost one all respect.[3] This North American compulsive drive for independence intensifies the threat of old age. The middle-aged do not want the elderly to encumber them and the elderly do not want to burden. Few of us, however, can avoid the awkwardness and dependencies of aging, since, as we are relentlessly told, the elderly are one minority which, sooner or later, almost all of us join.

THE PATTERNS OF CARE

This essay cannot cover the variety of medical troubles that beset the elderly. I will sketch, rather, the basic patterns for their care in the family, in homes of their own, and in total institutions, patterns which, however indispensable, place special moral demands upon them.

Family Care. No institution compares with the family in caring for the elderly. Seventy-five to eighty percent of the elderly have families nearby. Eighty percent have seen a family member in the last week. Of those not institutionalized, half live alone and half with relatives. The government informally subsidizes this family-centered care through indexed increases in Social Security payments that far exceed the pensioner's original contribution to the system. This regular source of income allows many older people to live for a time near their children or other relatives without becoming a full-time dependent. But our society does not subsidize adequately services that one finds in other countries: for example, respite houses where the elderly may go for brief periods of time that provide adult children in Great Britain with a break from constant care; or, home visitation services that permit more elderly to function independently and longer in the vicinity of their children.

The migration of large numbers of the elderly to the Sun Belt has led to the development of another kind of family care—the growth of extended families of the elderly who help one another. These families no longer depend upon their children to take care of them but upon older, "adopted" brothers and sisters, to take care of one another; some of them flourish a little better than others, but all of them are roughly in the same boat, in need of someone to play bridge with, talk to, or who monitors daily the window shade that signals whether all is well or disaster has struck during the night. This extended family functions within the limits of fragile resources and energies. Like the biological family, it relies on the reciprocities of giving and receiving and mutual dependency.

Within the bonds of family life, taking care of the elderly presupposes a network of giving and receiving, of mutual, though not simultaneous, dependency. We honor our fathers and mothers (and other elderly people within the family circle) because, at least in part, we have received so much from them—life itself, care and nurture, the investment of love (however inept it may have been), family history mediated through their deeds and stories, the mystery of our origins, and a hint of our destiny. The care we give therefore responds in part to the love that preceded it. The elderly are dependent now; and our caring for them answers in part to our original dependency upon them and in part to the dependency which we ourselves, one day, will face in old age.

Independent Living. Care beyond the family circle occurs usually within a different moral structure; chiefly, that of the marketplace. The ethical standards of buying and selling rather than giving and receiving control much professional care and nonprofessional service. The elderly who pride themselves on their independence usually in fact depend heavily on strangers. They rely on money to buy professional and nonprofessional services. They often prefer this impersonal dependency to the personal dependency within the family circle. They prefer to buy, or would seem to prefer to buy, the care, service, and attention of strangers.

(The Social Security system provides a major support for the freedom of the elderly to continue participating in the marketplace. We call Social Security an entitlement program, thus suggesting that the system returns to the elderly what they and their employers have contributed —plus interest. But in fact, until recently, the average worker has withdrawn much more from the system than he or she put into it; in the early 1980s, for example, a retired worker might take out in the first twenty-two months of retirement the $14,000 he would have deposited into the system across a lifetime. This fiction of entitlement has both a moral and a political advantage. Morally, it spares the elderly from having to subject themselves to an embarrassing "means test" to claim support. Politically, the well-nigh universal participation of rich and poor alike in the system guarantees it broad and sustained support. Unfortunately, this indiscriminate subsidy to rich and poor alike among the elderly has created a drain on the system. In a time of budgetary retrenchment, some reformers increasingly wondered whether it was fair to let entitlement programs for the elderly grow apace while the national administration cut poverty programs for mothers and children and others to the bone; some fiscal conservatives, on the other hand, wanted to cut benefits back to a level too low to support the modestly fixed. A fair compromise solution would subject one-half of a pensioner's Social Security income benefits to ordinary income tax rates. That percentage would roughly equal the employer's original contribution —which the government had not taxed—to the Social Security fund. The poor would not make enough from all sources to be taxed, and the rich would no longer claim untaxed windfall. Meanwhile, funds would increase to support basic income for the poor and the modestly fixed among the elderly without imposing an unsavory "means test").

Professional caregivers loom especially large in the life of the elderly, whether or not they live alone. An old *New Yorker* cartoon graphically illustrated this point by changing the relative size of significant others at different stages in a person's life. In childhood, the mother, of course, dominates. Then the father grows in scale. In youth, friends expand at the expense of mother and father until parents at length fade before a single romantic partner and mate. Co-workers and children fill the middle years but eventually diminish as the nest empties and the retirement dinners take place. When at length the mate sickens and dies, perhaps the doctor, the nurse, the lawyer, or, for some, a pastor figures prominently in the final scene. Exaggerated (since the data show heavy reliance on family members for care), but still the cartoon reminds us that in our advanced age the professional often offers security and sanctuary for a price. Appointments with the physician become red-letter days on the calendar around which time gets organized. How professionals treat the elderly acquires an even greater significance since professionals increasingly represent and symbolize for the elderly their treatment at the hands of the society at large.

Professionals, of course, vary greatly in their habits of respect for the elderly. Some intervene with a powerful sense of solidarity with

their patients and clients. Others condescend. The professional relationship itself inherently reflects a power imbalance between professionals
and clients, and tempts to condescension. This imbalance shows up
etymologically. The lawyer as "advocate," literally *speaks for* his client.
The word "client," on the other hand, means "auditor," that is, a troubled person who needs a mouthpiece working on his behalf. The word
"patient" similarly denotes passivity. The sick, triply passive, suffer the
ravages of disease, the heroic measures of the professional, and the aggressive action of drugs, knife, and laser beam in the body. This power
imbalance compounds, often quite automatically, as younger professionals deal with the elderly. Professionals of all stripes who handle the
infirm and the aged display their health and youth—often rather unwittingly—like a bustling cold front that moves in and stiffens the land-
scape.

Idealistic members of the helping professions do not easily avoid
estranging condescension. The professional ethical ideal of philanthropy
reflects and reinforces rather than redresses the original imbalance in
the relationship. The conscientious professional defines himself or herself as a relatively self-sufficient monad who draws on knowledge-based
power and bestows benefactions on clients. Clients appear before the
professional in their ignorance or their age, which the professional as
doctor, lawyer, social worker, nurse, minister, or teacher offers to rem-
edy. Idealistic professionals tend to define themselves as the benefactors,
the clients as relatively passive beneficiaries. Thus they tend to obscure
for themselves the degree to which professionals actually receive from
their clients not only money, but, in a sense, their vocation. This reci-
procity once obscured, a gulf opens between benefactor and beneficiary.
Philanthropy isolates. As Ronald Blythe put it, "The old do not want
outreach, they want association."[4]

Total Institutions. Eventually the day arrives when the elderly can
no longer participate directly in the marketplace, whether through their
own savings or through a third party payment system. The pattern of
solving the problem of care through buying and selling has already settled in, however. Now the need arises for purchasing a total environment of care for the elderly who can no longer care for themselves.
To that end, we mobilize professional and subprofessional services in
large institutions (the hospital, the retirement center, the nursing
home).

The strategy of placing the aged in large facilities springs from a
variety of motives, sometimes benevolent, at other times self-serving,
and often a mixture of both. In some cases the elderly flourish best
in total institutions, their alternatives are so limited. Either they have
no family or they require a level of care that their family (often composed
of another infirm or elderly person) can no longer provide. Most poign-

antly, in some cases the family would like to continue providing care but incontinence and/or senility make it impossible for the family to cope.

Still, a substantial minority of 20 to 30 percent of the residents in total institutions live there for reasons other than health or family circumstances.[5] They require more care than they previously received or knew how to secure in the outside world, but they do not really need the total institutional care facility. The segregation of such in hospitals and nursing homes reflects, in part, our tendency to medicalize the problem of aging. We provide for too few intermediate alternatives between independence, life in the family, and total institutional care. Often the delivery of a few strategic services would make independent or family life possible, and, of course, much cheaper than providing total service in an institution. The economics of our delivery system, however, favor institutionalization.

Statistically, the percentage of the elderly residing in nursing homes today seems inconsequential. About 5 to 6 percent live in such facilities. The statistics, however, mislead. Although at any given time only 6 percent of those over sixty-five live in a nursing home, 20 percent will spend some time, and many will die, there. Often the prospect shadows the last years of life. Moreover, I am convinced that those who *fear* ending up in a nursing home far exceed the percentage of those who spend some time there.

The nursing home occupies the same place in the psyche of the elderly today that the poorhouse and the orphanage played in the imagination of Victorian children. Even those who never set foot in such a facility fear it as fate.

The deprivations that total institutions impose hardly argue for dismantling them. They have their place. But planners must give serious thought to their design, particularly to what might be called the moral significance of "turf."

Before the twentieth century, physicians and nurses ordinarily came to the patient's home to deliver their services. Only the poor went to the hospital. Now rich and poor alike get transported to the professional's domain. The very architecture of the hospital and the nursing home tends to reflect and serve the convenience of the staff and the machines that dominate these institutions. Disease has already disabled the patient; now strange noises, rhythms, and procedures in the hospital further enfeeble and baffle. Uprooted from familiar settings where they felt in charge, patients must now surrender to the control of strangers. Not surprisingly, the elderly balk even more than the sick at entering total institutions. The immediate stakes are so much higher for the elderly. Sick people go to the hospital because they must, and they hope to come out alive. The elderly usually move to the retirement care center permanently and irreversibly. The center, for them, precedes and heralds death. The institution swallows them up; its limited room prevents them from bringing many of their valued possessions and other tokens of identity. The new location often removes them from the dwindling little community they knew. It often buries them prematurely.

Successively and progressively, impairment, old age, immobility, and death restrict space. The world at large diminishes to a single room and ultimately to a casket. Ordinarily people live in a number of different environments—home, workplace, streets, parks, gardens, and sidewalks. The bedroom serves as only part of a total world, often a sanctuary from it. But, for the immobile or the impaired, the world shrinks to a single room. Designers of total institutions take on an awesome responsibility. They create for residents not just a fragment but the whole of their world. Meanwhile, the psychic life of the elderly also implodes into a preoccupation with the body and its troubles. Both physical space and psychic space contract. The design of humane institutions for the elderly requires sensitive reflection on the older person's perception of his or her body and the contracting world it inhabits.

In the introduction to this book I talked about the threefold service of the body to a human being: it helps us control and savor the world and it serves as the medium for revealing oneself. The elderly suffer loss in each of these services. Illness and aging already steal some control. Moving into a facility can further diminish control, not only because the elderly person moves to another's turf, but also because the shock of the move can assault the memory and, with it, the capacity to function. A man in his eighties living alone and long familiar with his surroundings may care for himself competently despite a tattered memory. He turns off the gas jet seven or eight times after preparing his breakfast. He has enough memory left to know that he should turn off the gas but not enough left to know whether he has done it. If, however, the society denies this man enough supplementary services to sustain him in familiar surroundings and places him in a large institution with its architectural accommodation to staff rather than to residents, then his memory and competence can precipitously deteriorate. Sensitive institutional design alone will not eliminate such problems, but it should attempt to reduce to a minimum the loss of control and the humiliation over that loss.

Bodies also supply us with the means to savor the world—far beyond the reach of our controlling. A home for the elderly substitutes a functionally bland environment for the variegated texture of the world that each of us has come to savor. (Yeats once complained about the formula H_2O: "I like a little seaweed in my definition of water.") Conscientious planners usually work hard to purge their buildings of the unpleasant smells that go with illness and old age. They also need to admit into the room/world of the elderly a few of the bona fides of sensuous life.

Finally, the body serves as a means to reveal ourselves to others. Separate me from my body and you divorce me from my community. In old age this separation increasingly occurs, and in two ways. In some cases the mind remains alert but the body sinks into ruin beneath it; in others, the body persists plausibly itself, but the mind abandons it. In the first instance, the alert feel their bodily defects less as imperfections than as stigmas. Indeed, since we *are* our bodies, the defects stigmatize not just the flesh but the whole person. Envy of the angels can tempt the obese adolescent and the elderly. One would like to escape from the body and its encumbrances altogether. One's body, and therefore one's self, no longer feels lovable, touchable, huggable, cherishable. This deprivation has its implications for institutional design. It calls for respect for the body, respect for modesty, even the modesty of the demented. And it reinforces the warrants for creating an attractive environment.

Rooms function as a kind of extension of our bodies. People find the bedridden more approachable if the room they inhabit is attractive. It casts a sacramental aura. The peculiar slant of sunlight, the texture of a rug, and the comfort of a chair become means of sharing. When the elderly offer a chair to a visitor, in a limited way they offer and extend themselves.

Recently built retirement centers have shown more sensitivity to the importance of physical surroundings. The elderly among the financially secure can enjoy a vastly improved institutional and communal life in the new, three-tiered, continuing-care retirement centers. They offer, according to capacity and need, for those who can pay for it, a graduated set of buildings from "independent living," through "assisted living," to "skilled nursing." Many of the facilities are physically appealing and well staffed. But the poor and the modestly fixed among the elderly cannot hope to enter them. "Continuing care retirement communities are within the financial reach of about 50 percent of the elderly. They are not an option for the less affluent," observes *Consumer Reports* in a sobering account of "What's Available for the Poor."[6] The Reagan administration "gutted" support for the successful and relatively scandal-free 202 program, reducing new housing units from 25,000 to 8,000 per year, substituting inferior construction materials for the earlier brick and masonry buildings, shrinking both personal and communal space in each building, and bypassing, where possible, the installation of such safety features as sprinkler systems and elevators. This deterioration of the infrastructure of institutional care for the elderly will eventually exact a high cost. Inferior buildings will require earlier and more costly repairs. And the lack of coordinate support services through the Department of Health and Human Services for 202 type facilities will drive the elderly into nursing homes much earlier and at a much higher cost per person each year.

THE VIRTUES AND VICES
OF THE ELDERLY

Moralists have concentrated on the ethics of caregivers but not on the ethics of care-receivers, except to emphasize the importance of granting patients and clients their personal autonomy. Ethicists, however, do not adequately respect the moral dignity of elderly (or other) patients if they simply clear out for them a zone of empty liberty while remaining indifferent to its particular uses. Ronald Blythe undercuts this condescending sentimentality in *The View in Winter*:

> Perhaps with full-span lives the norm, people may have to learn how to be aged as they once had to learn to be adult. It may soon be necessary and legitimate to criticise the long years of vapidity in which a healthy elderly person does little more than eat and play bingo, or who consumes excessive amounts of drugs, or who expects a self-indulgent stupidity to go unchecked. Just as the old should be convinced that whatever happens during senescence, they will never suffer exclusion, so they should understand that age does not exempt them from being despicable.
>
> . . . .
>
> One of the most dreadful sights in the country of the old is that of the long rows of women playing the Las Vegas slot machines. Had Dante heard of it he would have cleared a space for it in hell.[7]

Blythe's scolding comment about the vices of some of the elderly —gluttony, pill-popping excess, compulsive gambling, prodigal wastes of time and money, and self-indulgent stupidity—should not mislead about the book he has written that movingly depicts the lives of the elderly in an English village. Rigorous moral criticism of the elderly does not inevitably remove them from human community. Quite the contrary: the failure to criticize the elderly and other like groups may subtly remove them from the human race.

So the Christian ethicist John Yoder argued in his *Politics of Jesus*. At first glance, the New Testament appears conservative in its discussion of the duties of husband and wives, parents and children, masters and slaves. The *Haustafeln* emphasizes the duties, rather than the rights, of the subordinate in each pair. But, in fact, the New Testament table of duties had a revolutionary potential in that it addressed *both* persons in the pair as moral agents. In this respect, the New Testament writers broke with the Stoic tables of domestic duties, which addressed only the person in a superior position, as though only the more powerful had a moral existence. But in the New Testament, "The *subordinate* person in the social order is *addressed as a moral agent*."[8] Hellenistic thought, Yoder argues, provided no other precedent for this revolutionary shift in attention. In addressing wives, children, and slaves, Christian scripture assigned "*personal* moral responsibility to those who have no legal or moral status in their culture, and makes of them decision-makers."[9] Western culture (and the church) took a long time catching up with this change of status. Not until the twentieth century did servants appear as more than comic figures in Western tragedy. Until still more recently, blacks and the elderly appeared as comic figures only, not to be taken seriously.

The neglect of the elderly as morally serious persons springs partly from our reduction of ethics to purely pragmatic issues of problem-solving. At the onset of this volume, I suggested that moral challenges include not only problems that we can pragmatically solve but also existential issues that admit of no solution but raise questions of our own self-definition. The appropriate question we face is not "What are we going to do about it?" but "How does one rise to the occasion?" The elderly, of course, face problems at both levels. The event of retirement, the onset of arthritis, flagging energies, the heart attack, the stroke, the death of a mate, the loss of beauty or verbal command, the shift from independent living into the family or into the total institution—such reversals demand pragmatic responses. They pose a series of problems to solve. But at a deeper level these challenges confront the elderly not simply with something to do, but with someone to be.

None of this self-definition comes easily. Inevitably, the elderly must contend with adversity. In response, the elderly need, of course, virtues or strengths of character. Virtues refer not only to those habits whereby we must transform our world through our deeds but also to those specific strengths that grow partly in response to adversities and sustain us in the midst of them.

Such virtues hardly come automatically with growing old. Even limited dealings with the elderly quickly disabuse us of that sentimentality. Rather, the virtues come only with resolution, struggle, perhaps prayer, and perseverance. Further, these virtues hardly appear only in the elderly. Some common human virtues—which men and women of all ages might do well to cultivate—simply take special form in the later years. When they do appear in the elderly, however, they can instruct and sometimes even inspire. Their example can particularly encourage the stricken and fainthearted among the young who associate the possibility of a human existence only under the accident of their own temporary flourishing.

The following sketch of the virtues deals only in passing and by implication with the vices. The too brief treatment of the vices runs the danger of adding to hurtful confusion. People often confuse physical infirmity with moral failing. When does the older person suffer from brain atrophy and when does he or she merely impose on others a self-indulgent stupidity? When does the old man betray the garrulousness

of the self-important bore, and when a driven verbal incontinence? In
the following, I have in mind not infirmities but vices; we only add
to the suffering of the infirm when we confuse the two.

Courage ranks first on the list of virtues. Westerners too often restrict
this virtue to the battlefield. But the soldier's prospect of death is uncertain; his separation from his loved ones but temporary. Not so for the
aged who face the certainty of imminent death and whose losses are
anything but temporary. Thomas Aquinas defined courage as a firmness
of soul in the face of adversity. That firmness may show itself far from
the battlefield. An eighty-year-old unmarried woman faces resolutely
her declining years; a widower suddenly takes his first steps alone after
fifty years of marriage; an aged mother finds her children too busy
to have her around. Courage does not presuppose fearlessness, a life
free of aversions; rather, it requires keeping one's fears, one's dislikes,
one's laziness under control for the sake of *the* good as well as for the
sake of one's own good.

Thomas Aquinas recognized two forms of courage: passive endurance and active attack. Courage in the elderly does not restrict itself
to endurance. Sociologist David Gutman has noted that the extremely
old survivor often evinces a feisty combativeness.[10]

Sometimes this combativeness can (and ought to) carry beyond private life into the political arena. Heroes among the elderly include the
old New Dealer Claude Pepper and the intrepid Gray Panther Maggie
Kuhn. In a nation given to interest-group politics, the elderly qualify
as one of those interest groups whose needs the society ought to meet;
they have a right to organize and to press for their interests.

Yet a democratic society cannot flourish if interest groups within
it fail to see themselves not only as interest groups but also as publics
within the larger public. What the Revolutionary thinkers called *public
virtue*, that is, a readiness to make some sacrifices for the common good,
distinguishes a public from a mere interest group. The Revolutionary
thinkers saw public virtue as characterizing the very soul of a republic.
Admittedly, only a naive idealism would expect any and all groups to
detach themselves wholly from questions of self-interest. Indeed, a republic requires that groups within it make their interests known, since
such subgroups—the elderly included—can usually determine their
own interests more accurately than can remote authority. At the same
time, one must pursue not simply one's own good but the common
good. Ironically, an intemperate pursuit of self-interest, unqualified by
considerations of the common good, eventually diminishes the stock
of those public goods (such as libraries, concerts, safe-ways for pedestri-
ans, parks, and gardens) upon which all people, the elderly particularly,
depend. Further, the unqualified pursuit of self-interest by the elderly
can impose injustice on other groups in dire need who do not have

the limited good fortune, in this case, of being old. Clearly, entitlement programs based on age alone can take away some resources desperately required by the needy whatever their age and may diminish the amounts available to the penurious among the elderly. The elderly should not submit themselves to the test of the common good alone, but neither should they exempt themselves from the obligation to public virtue.

Humility. Most people at sixty-five can look forward to a dozen years of good health; some, much more. Most people require substantial care in the last six months to a year of their lives. They depend upon the virtue of love or benevolence in their caregivers.[11] At the same time, the elderly find themselves in the awkward position of being receivers. While it may be more blessed to give than to receive, it can be considerably more uncomfortable to receive than to give. The virtue of *humility*, necessary to receivers in human life, does not come easily, especially to Americans, who take pride in their independence and their giving. Yet the progressive loss of friends, job, bodily prowess, and energy, the passing look on the face of the young that tells us we are old, these experiences assault one's dignity; they humiliate. All the care in the world will not overcome the sting of humiliation; only humility can. It bears remembering that the words for human, humility, and earth itself—humus—have the same root. God took the dust of the earth and breathed his spirit upon it and brought men and women into being: human, humus, beset by humiliation but destined for humility. Perhaps mid-life would not be so scary, so spoiled by pretension, so shadowed by the fear of failure and the dread of dependence, if we knew how to keep our feet in the soil of humility, to not be so afraid of the soil to which we shall return.

Patience does not inevitably characterize old age; advancing years and infirmity provoke anger, frustration, and bitterness. The virtue, moreover, trivializes when we interpret it as a state of pure passivity. Patience requires purposive waiting, receiving, willing; it demands a most intense sort of activity; it requires taking control of one's spirit precisely when all else goes out of control, when panic would send us sprawling in all directions. Such patience calls for a resolute activity deeper than that frenzied state of busyness that characterizes mid-life. Most people live out their middle years in a state of passive activity. Despite the appearance of great activity, their agendas are really set by the drift of things: the demands of others, the volume of work to be done, the day's schedule to keep up with. They tend to go on automatic pilot, which gives but the illusion of a great and heroic purposefulness. But sickness, sudden loss, protracted pain, the curtailed movement of old age, bring all this bustling to a halt and require that the elderly find their bearings as purposive beings.

The Benedictine monks used to talk about other marks—moral marks—of old age: *simplicitas* and *benignitas*.[12]

Simplicity should mark the elderly, and not merely because memory lapses into its familiar, repetitive grooves, but because the pilgrim has at long last learned how to travel light. He has learned to live by simple truths and simple gifts. The prophet Micah describes such a soul as it winnows down, unencumbered, toward that purity of heart which wills one thing.

> With what shall I come before the Lord, and bow myself before God on high? Shall I come before him with burnt offerings, with calves a year old? Will the Lord be pleased with thousands of rams, with ten thousands of rivers of oil? Shall I give my first-born for my transgression, the fruit of my body for the sin of my soul? He has showed you, O man, what is good; and what does the Lord require of you but to do justice, and to love kindness, and to walk humbly with your god? (Micah 6:6–8.)

Old age hardly produces automatically the virtue of *benignity*, which the monks understood as a kind of purified benevolence. Quite the contrary, the *ars moriendi* of the late Middle Ages identified avarice as the chief besetting sin of the aged. The closer one gets to the final dispossession of death, the more fiercely one may seek to clutch one's possessions, holding, grasping, managing, manipulating. The hands have always symbolized the sin of avarice. It tempts those for whom insecurity is maximal, and mobility, except for the reach of the hands, minimal. Benevolence opposes the tightfistedness of avarice, not with the empty-handedness of death but with the open-handedness of love.

Integrity. Some thinkers link—and I believe rightly—the virtue of integrity with an inclusive unity of character rather than interpret the virtue as a part of the whole. Since a moral structure rather than a mere temperamental state defines character as a whole, one needs, in addition to all particular virtues, a virtue that summarizes and includes that inclusive structure. Like all other virtues, integrity must be acquired rather than result from disposition alone or from an automatic ripening that age guarantees.

Integrity draws on the overlapping images of uprightness and wholeness. The image of uprightness reminds us that integrity has to do with moral posture—the perpendicular. It does not stoop to conquer. Earlier life tests one's integrity in the forward scramble for admission to privileged schools and in the competition for grades, position, approval, and neighborhood. The upright professional refuses to put his nose to the ground, sniffing out opportunities at the expense of clients, customers, and colleagues, or bowing before the powerful, or knuckling under external pressure.

Uprightness, in one sense, comes more easily in old age. The years of warping ambition have passed. A more powerful generation no longer lies ahead to intimidate and reward. The George Bernard Shaws, the Harold Ickes, and the Maggie Kuhns symbolize an intrepid and upright old age, articulate and well-nigh fearless. Yet old age *per se* hardly bestows that uprightness. Some elderly, to be sure, feel freer to speak out, less frightened than formerly of the opinion and reaction of others. But a person had best develop some measure of probity during the earlier years when the rewards for obsequiousness abound. The opinionated garrulousness of some elderly compensates for years of verbal servitude; it does not reflect the uprightness of integrity.

The virtue also signifies a wholeness or completeness of character, a roundedness, as it were, a self gathered up into a unity, not scattered or dispersed. Such wholeness of character does not permit a division or split between the inner and the outer, between word and deed. In this respect, the image overlaps with uprightness. Integrity makes possible the bond of trust between human beings. Integral persons, undivided and upright, do not say one thing while intending another. At one with themselves, they do not need to dissemble with others or deceive themselves.

No one recognized better than Augustine of Hippo that integrity's rounded completion of the self does not come automatically with aging. His *Confessions*—often called the first autobiography written in the West —deliberately retrieved and re-presented Augustine's own past not for the sake of vain self-preoccupation but as part of a mystic discipline. He needed to engage in a steadfast, often painful retrieval of the self out of its scattered, dispersed, and squandered state to make possible its ascent to the divine. In Augustine's perspective, no self yet exists to commune with God without this re-collection, this integration, as it were; and this re-collection itself cannot take place, fully and freely, without the conviction of the forgiveness of sins. Forgiveness alone lets one come to terms wholly with one's past; it frees the confessor from the need to engage in fancy ploys to impress others or from even fancier self-deception.

Some modern people, of course, see a partial and secular analogue to this religious recovery of wholeness in the discipline of psychoanalysis, which requires a painful retrieval of the past in the course of a final self-recovery. Those who cannot afford the luxury of such formal analysis must find their own makeshift ways of binding up their lives and healing memory. Thus, the elderly informally engage in the moral work of autobiography.

Gone wrong, this life review[13] deteriorates into a melancholic nostalgia, a profitless, endlessly repetitive and wistful reliving of the past, or a remorseful, sometimes bitter, invocation of ghosts. More constructively, it signals the aspiration for a completed life, where the ending rounds a corner and recovers the beginning. Fittingly, the analyst Erik Erikson defines integrity as "accrued ego integration,"[14] more broadly as the integration of the self with its social, cultural, and ethnic heritage. A religious echo sounds in the few sentences Erikson wrote on the subject. He recognizes that wholeness—especially in the elderly—requires a reckoning with fate and death: fate accepted "as the frame of life," death "as its finite boundary."[15] Fate and death test the virtue because they constantly threaten the self with its dispossession; they would leave it empty rather than full. They oppress the self with what it has failed to accomplish or with the triviality of its accomplishments; they turn all goods to ashes and disconnect the self from all its previously accepted meanings. Thus disgust and despair beset the self and unravel all its petty integrations.

In Erikson's judgment, the virtue of integrity alone, *qua* virtue, can hardly tame death and reduce it to the relatively quiescent boundary of human existence. Rather, death looms as the abyss that confounds all provisional meanings—unless the event can be set within the context of a transcendent meaning. Thus Erikson had to close his discussion of the virtue by linking the moral with the religious. He invokes the Tillichian phrase "ultimate concerns," and closes his discussion of integrity and old age with a passing reference to the "great philosophical and religious systems."[16]

Many will shy away from this attempt to link integrity with religious conviction, and certainly with the explicitly theological. But even our ordinary sense of the word "integrity" presses beyond the purely self-referential and toward a standard that transcends the self. We instinctively recognize that a man has lost his integrity when his identity with that ultimate aim and purpose that grounded his life breaks asunder. The completeness or roundedness of integrity differs from mere personal self-sufficiency. While referring to the self in its wholeness, integrity also points beyond the self toward the person, the ideal, the transcendent, which gives shape to the person's life. The virtue refers to the inclusive self, to be sure, but the self turns out to be ecstatic —pitched out beyond itself toward that in which it finds its meaning.

Most people, as indicated in the introduction, connect with the transcendent or express their ultimate concerns chiefly through rituals. These rituals may derive partly from official religious traditions, but they also include those repeated actions in daily life that signal both one's chief worries and one's ultimate resources. We often dismiss these actions as "routines," but routines in rising, bathing, preparing food, shopping, reading, monitoring TV, receiving a visitor, signaling a neighbor, and securing an apartment at night tell us a lot about how a person deals with anxiety, boredom, fear, and loneliness and what resources or lack of them shape his or her life.

On the whole, older women seem to sustain more successfully than elderly men the moral/ritual side of life. Caregivers notice that widows often lead "fuller lives" than widowers. Old men are much more likely, once having retired, lost a mate, or suffered a reduction in income, to withdraw or to allow their lives to dwindle to a minimal routine. Men shrink more readily than women to an abstract cipher, disconnected and noncommunicative.

Many reasons suggest themselves for these contrasting "performances" of older men and women. To some it seems providential that women, who are biologically fated to live longer than men, adjust better than men to old age. Women also receive an earlier biological preview of aging, if not of mortality—menopause gives them a clearer signal about the life cycle—whereas men often fail to decipher whatever signals they receive. Women tend more than men to associate aging and death with the corruption of bodily form; men, with a flagging vitality. The corruption of the body shows up relentlessly in the morning mirror; the failure of vitality overtakes more elusively, and men suppress it more easily—although a poet like Eliot dispatches an entire civilization under the symbol of failing male power, "I am an old man in a dry month."

The sexes have differed until recently in a still further way that affects later performance. When the nest emptied, a woman, while still in her middle years, needed to face and adjust to the loss of her major vocation. A man did not suffer that trauma until much later, at retirement, when his resources and resilience may have declined. Middle-class and professional men sought their life's meaning in and through the unilinear progression of a career. Once detached from that career, life lost its tang. Compensatory routines smacked of the trivial. Men who chronically complained about the corporation while they worked for it nevertheless prized retrospectively their identity with it. Upon retirement, they found it more difficult than women to body forth their life in rituals, more cyclical than unilinear in their justifying source. Divorced from work, men find themselves harder put to develop fitting habits of friendship, love, food, conversation, art, celebration, and play. They find it much more difficult than women to achieve, display, and share the rounded, full, and connected life integrity creates.

The massive shift since World War II of women into the outside workforce will doubtless change this cultural contrast. A majority of women, like men, will now face a major adjustment at a much later age when coping grows more difficult and a new life and structure become harder to mount. We are much too close to these changes to assess long-range consequences, but until recently, the contrasts in ritual life have been striking.

Conventional wisdom emphasizes *wisdom* as a special virtue of the elderly. Age brings with it accrual of experience, and, to the degree that one learns from experience, one gains wisdom—so older politicians have always proclaimed as they run for reelection. The related practical virtue of *prudence*, as the medieval moralists analyzed it, makes integrity possible.

Prudence included three parts: *memoria, docilitas,* and *solertia.*

Memoria characterizes the person who remains open to his or her past, without retouching, falsifying, or glorifying it. Such openness, as we have seen, makes possible the wholeness of integrity. But *memoria* should not be confused with the propensity of many elderly folk to wander endlessly in Yesterday. Old age hardly offers *memoria* automatically. Indeed, it especially tempts to the falsifications of nostalgia and remorse.

Docilitas connotes not the passivity of the English word "docility," but a capacity to perceive the present—alertness, an attentiveness in the moment. *Docilitas* signifies a capacity to be silent, to be still, and thus to perceive. It helps keep the elderly connected to others. Garrulity in old age sadly deprives old men and women of the present and the presence of others.

Solertia completes, if you will, the threefold temporal ecstasy of prudence. It signifies a readiness for the unexpected. Once again, old age hardly guarantees such openness toward the future. On the contrary, the lives of many older people harden into routines which make the unexpected always unwelcome. Yet rigidity does not entirely define the elderly. Sometimes, they do learn how to "travel light." They learn to sit loose, as it were, on life, more so than the beleaguered middle-aged. The event of death, of course, symbolizes everything contingent and unexpected about the future. While death is certain, its time is not. (By way of emphasizing the uncontrollable intrusiveness of death, Muriel Spark, in *Memento Mori,* her novel about the residents of a nursing home, lets death intrude by a telephone call.) Readiness for the unexpected includes a readiness for death. The elderly at their best teach us that.

Erik Erikson links the traditional virtue of wisdom with detachment, which depends in part upon a store of experience. The inexperienced are prone to overreact or underreact. They do not know how to weigh and evaluate what has happened to them. They are inclined to let a catastrophe engulf them or to overinvest in particular goods or outcomes. They do not yet know how to worry wisely or to love wisely. (For this reason, grandparents often seem wiser than their adult children in relating to the next generation. Parents are inclined to drive their own ambitions like a long stake through their children. Grandparents seem a little more detached and freer to enjoy and savor without bending the young to the warp of their own frustrated hopes.)

But one must not confuse detachment with the Stoic ideal of the passionless state. The Stoic ideal of apathy solved the problem of suffering by banking low the fires of desire. The Stoics urged the self to operate at the lowest possible wattage—to keep lit, at most, a nightlight. Such a self suffers little because it risks little and loves not at all. It detaches itself from any and all things before the final extinction of death. The Stoic ideal evinced its own dignity in kings and slaves alike; it depended upon a rare, almost aristocratic, rational self-control and discipline. In the modern world, some managers of the elderly in institutions impose on residents a mockery of such detachment. They want their residents relatively passive, compliant, laid back, and yielding. They can manage the very old more easily if they are doped up, unobtrusive, unintrusive, and dozing. The Stoic argued for a clear-headed detachment; the unscrupulous manager reduces the elderly to the apathy of the vegetable.

The biblical tradition defines the virtue of wisdom differently than does the Stoic.[17] The biblical tradition achieves perspective on the human condition not through an all-encompassing detachment but through a primordial attachment. In the setting of Christianity, this fundamental attachment to the divine love sustains, but also orders and limits, all other attachments and fears. It produces two virtues, which, for want of better terms, we might designate as Christian nonchalance and Christian courtesy. (I should not call them Christian virtues—for the obvious reason that other than Christians evince them. But it may be of some general interest to indicate the specifically Christian warrants for them.) Both virtues spring from serenity—a metaphysical serenity in the case of nonchalance and a social serenity in the case of courtesy. Nonchalance reveals a capacity to take in one's stride life's gifts and blows; courtesy, a comparable capacity to deal honorably with all that is urgent, jarring, and rancorous on the social scene.

Neither virtue, at least as enjoined in the religious tradition at its best, urges passivity. They are virtues for pilgrims—those who are in but not of the world, those who know how to sit loose to the world. The virtues hardly invite an unattached indifference. Indeed, not a Christian quietist, but the politically active, prophetic theologian Reinhold Niebuhr recommended, in his later years, Romans 8 as the *classicus locus* for a Christian nonchalance. The passage does not, in the fashion of Christian Science or secular versions of optimism, solve the problem of suffering by denying the reality of disease, pain, aging, and death; it puts these destructive forces in the setting of a power that persists and endures in the midst of them. God ultimately encompasses the powers that dazzle and terrorize the heart; they are *real* but not *ultimate*; these powers do not speak the last word about the human condition,

> neither death, nor life, nor angels, nor principalities, nor things present, nor things to come, nor powers, nor height, nor depth, nor anything else in all creation, will be able to separate us from the love of God. (Romans 8:38–39)

The Apostle Paul does not ground this nonchalance in a Stoic detachment, a final state of apathy that conveniently settles on the heart precisely at that late moment in life when the fires of desire seem to flicker and gutter. For the divine love which justifies nonchalance did not avoid or eliminate suffering and death, but itself experienced the full range of human need. However, it exposes the final inability of tribulation and death to separate men and women from God. Located within the dynamics of the divine love, the self can begin to sit loose to the world. It can meet its obligations within the world without panicking before it or getting mired in it.

This metaphysical nonchalance leads to the social virtue of courtesy. Ties to others can deepen precisely because they have been lightened. A primordial tie makes other ties bearable. Men and women can see the needs of others and their own in a more spacious setting that makes courtesy in the midst of pain, aging, suffering, and dying possible.

This more spacious setting makes sense of a final virtue which the Benedictine monks associated with old age, *hilaritas*. At first glance, hilarity seems out of place in the elderly. In fact, they are more clinically disposed than their juniors to depression. Anxiety over resources, grief over loss, insufficient exercise, broken sleep patterns, and diminished appetites precede and accompany depression. Yet the monks talk about *hilaritas*, a kind of celestial gaiety in those who have seen a lot, done a lot, grieved a lot, but now acquire that humored detachment of the fly on the ceiling looking down on the human scene.

Whatever special meaning hilarity may have for monks in the monastery, they hardly possess it alone. Children are blessed when their grandparents' lightness of spirit offers sunny relief from their parents' gravity.

The year before his death, Yeats expressed this hilarity in *Lapis Lazuli*, a poem that spreads out the whole human scene of "old civilizations put to the sword":

> Two Chinamen, behind them a third,
> Are carved in lapis lazuli,
> Over them flies a long-legged bird,
> A symbol of longevity;
> The third, doubtless a serving man,

The third, doubtless a serving man,
Carries a musical instrument.

Every discoloration of the stone,
Every accidental crack or dent,
Seems a water-course or an avalanche,
Or lofty slope where it still snows
Though doubtless plum or cherry-branch
Sweetens the little half-way house
These Chinamen climb towards, and I
Delight to imagine them seated there;
There, on the mountain and the sky,
On all the tragic scene they stare.
One asks for mournful melodies;
Accomplished fingers begin to play.
Their eyes mid many wrinkles, their eyes,
Their ancient glittering eyes, are gay.[18]

AFFLICTING THE AFFLICTED
Total Institutions

THIS CHAPTER WILL examine institutions as symbols of death, not those institutions and movements that obviously traffic in killing—war, concentration camps, revolutionary terrorism—but rather our health care institutions, which, though devoted to the fight against death, often become its instrument and symbol. Our total institutions reflect primordial images for sickness and death, images of hiding and devouring prominent in folklore, literature, dream life, and ritual behavior.[1]

Traditional societies interpreted sickness as the soul's departure from the body; and death as the soul's irreversible journey to a hidden realm. The enfeebled condition of the sick man or woman suggested that the animating principle, that is, the soul, had obviously vacated the body and retired to an invisible place, inaccessible to ordinary folk. Only the shaman could heal by tracking after and retrieving the soul, a feat which the healer accomplished by going into an ecstatic trance. He left his own body to fetch back the soul of the afflicted.

On death, when, at length, the soul departed for good, the body of the deceased turned into a shroud, a mask; that is, it now hid rather than revealed the soul that once animated it. Fittingly, funeral rites must shroud the shroud, that is, wrap up the body, and hide it away permanently in the ground. This final ritual of hiding carried the weight of a religious duty with which none could interfere. Thus Sophocles' King Creon horrified Antigone by refusing to let her bury her traitorous brother's body. No crime could place a man's body beyond the dignity of burial. Polyneices' corpse should not remain exposed to view where men could stare at it. Antigone had an indefectible duty to hide it from sight.

Sickness and death additionally suggest the image of devouring. To this day, we associate some diseases with eating. We call tuberculosis "consumption"; the malignant tumor feeds off its host; high fever burns and consumes. "Eating, devouring, hunger, death, and maw go together," writes Erich Neumann, "and we still speak, just like the primitive, of 'death's maw,' a 'devouring war,' a 'consuming disease.' "[2]

TOTAL INSTITUTIONS AND
THE TEMPTATION TO HIDE THE SICK,
THE AGED, THE IMPRISONED,
AND THE MENTALLY ILL

Increasingly, in the modern world, we have placed the sick, the aged, the criminal, and the mentally impaired and disturbed in total institutions, thereby segregating them from the society at large. Some 80 percent of Americans will eventually die not in the home, but in a total institution. The nursing home industry has expanded rapidly in recent decades, and special regions of the country have turned into huge territorial nursing homes where we hide the aged and they hide from us. It used to be said that children should be seen but not heard. Now we imply to many of the aged that they should be neither seen nor heard. Long before their death, we bury them in the folds of the total institution, hidden, out of sight and out of mind, until we are called upon, finally, to bury them again.

Similarly, mental hospitals and penal institutions subliminally associate with the oblivion of death. "'The prisoner,' a Sing Sing chaplain observed, 'was taught to consider himself dead to all without the prison walls.'"[3] A warden in 1826 prohibited contacts with the outside world, saying, "while confined here . . . you are to be literally buried from the world."[4] Such strictures on communication with the outside world have lessened today, but, still, prisoners call themselves the forgotten men. Our society has insisted on the thick walls of prisons and other institutions not only to keep inmates in but also to keep the world out. The walls say two things to an inmate: do not expect to *escape* from here, but also do not really expect others to visit you here. The society preaches the same message to many of the mentally disturbed and the chronically ill when it consigns them to institutional bins where they sometimes receive minimal, custodial care until their final disappearance.

This colonization of the distressed occurs for all the understandable reasons that obtain in a highly differentiated society with its specialized functions and services. The seriously distressed or disabled often overload the already burdened nuclear family. American society has not offered enough assists to family caregivers to provide them with some respite and relief. Institutions, moreover, can deliver important technical services that only mobilized professional resources can offer. I am not a Luddite who would urge that we smash the bureaucracies, that we "total" the total institutions or recklessly "deinstitutionalize" their residents. When we cast out the mentally disturbed from the huge custodial institutions where they were formerly incarcerated and recolonize them in third-rate hotels unattended, they go off their medication and end up in the streets. The heartless 1980s made that clear.

Yet we need to acknowledge candidly the suffering that our efforts to heal impose, the ordeals which the residents of our institutions face, partly gratuitous and eliminable, partly ineradicable, if we would offer what we can compassionately and effectively.

Some nursing homes have provided particularly cynical, even scandalous care; the mentally disturbed often receive notoriously poor treatment of their physical ailments. One harassed hospital administrator in New York City spoke with particular bitterness: apparently, he said, the emotionally disturbed are miraculously endowed with immunity to disease once committed to a mental hospital. For, in the New York City hospitals with which he is familiar, the insane never seem to come down with cancer, gall bladder trouble, or pulmonary or heart conditions serious enough to treat.

Although such neglect is remediable, institutionalization, whether good or bad, often tends to afflict the afflicted more subtly, by depriving them of community. The existentialists used to define being human as "being present" to others and letting others be present to oneself. Institutionalization often not only deprives the inmate of the opportunity to be present to the community but also relieves the larger society of the need to be present to the aged and distressed.

Although one would not want to do without the technical services that our health bureaucracies offer, they can exact a high price by imposing upon residents a kind of premature burial. The institution forces upon them a loss of name, identity, companionship, and acclaim—an extremity of deprivation of which the ordinary citizen has a foretaste in his complaints about the anonymous and impersonal conditions of modern life. To this degree, the nursing home for the poor, the prison, and the chronic care hospital serve as destination and symbol for a society at large that already operates to deprive its citizens of significance. Many people have suffered a loss of community long before their institutionalization. Indeed, the institution may in fact provide them with more community than they have enjoyed for years.

THE HOSPITAL AND DEATH
AS DEVOURER

While disease wracks his body, the acutely ill patient often has a more general sense of being exhausted and consumed by a world that has depleted all his personal resources. In the recent Western past, when a member of the middle class suffered a breakdown in health he sought respite in the sanctuary of the home, where the doctor visited him. This pattern of care prevailed for the middle and upper classes through the nineteenth and early twentieth centuries. Treatment for the poor differed. The poor went to the teaching hospitals, where, in exchange for medical services, they sometimes signed over to the staff their cadavers for research purposes. Thus the hospital acquired, especially for the poor, associations as an institution that not only serves, but consumes the body.

Today, care for the seriously ill among the middle and upper classes has moved to the hospitals, thus giving other members of society a taste of the earlier plight of the indigent. Despite its indisputable technological advantages over the home, the hospital exacts a high price both psychologically and financially. Psychologically, it gnaws—with its alien machines, rhythms, language, and routines—at that identity which a person previously maintained in the outside world. The patient must surrender his customary *control* of his world not only to the disease but to those who fight against it. His capacity for *savoring* his world is also numbed by the disease and by those procedures imposed upon him in the fight against it—diet, drugs, X-rays, surgery, nausea-inducing therapy, and sleeping potions. Finally, his capacity for *communicating* with his world erodes as he loses his social role. Just as disease rips him out of his usual place in the community and makes him feel less secure in his dealings with fellows, the procedures of the hospital remind him acutely of this loss by placing him in the hands of professionals—the nurse and the doctor—precisely those who seem unassailably secure in their own identities.

The financial trauma patients face makes it difficult to think of the hospital as sanctuary. Not only disease but medical expenses devour the patient, and if not the patient, the patient's family. Current systems of national health care, while distributing costs somewhat, have caused the total social expense of medicine to rocket to nearly 12 percent of the gross national product without increasing commensurately, as compared with other developed nations, the quality of health care. Nothing quite matches inflation for producing a sense that one's world is a devouring world; and no item has matched health care in the inventory of rising costs.

Chronic, even more than acute, care centers have acquired associations with death as devourer. Erving Goffman has worked out this theme in his long essay on asylums, a term which covers prisons, mental hospitals, monasteries, and the like, places where "a large number of like-situated individuals, cut off from the wider society for an appreciable period of time, together lead an enclosed, formally administered round of life."[5] Such an institution devours in the sense that it can deprive systematically the sick, the deviant, and the aged of their former identities.

> The recruit comes into the establishment with a conception of himself made possible by certain stable social arrangements in his home world. Upon entrance, he is immediately stripped of the support provided by these arrangements. In the accurate language of some of our oldest institutions, he begins a series of abasements, degradations, humiliations, and profanations of self. His self is systematically, if often unintentionally, mortified. . . .[6]

Goffman particularly attends to admission rites and procedures. The act of taking off one's old clothes and donning new garments impresses symbolically upon the inmate the price he must pay for entering into the total institution: the surrender of his old personal identity and autonomy and the acquisition of a new identity oriented to the authority of the professional staff and to the aims and purposes and the smooth operation of the institution. (The metaphor of changing clothes, of course, dates all the way back to the Benedictine Rule, and behind that to the letters of the Apostle Paul, and, still earlier, to rites of passage in primitive societies. It tells the prospective candidate that his new life demands devouring of the old, though in the case of the asylum inmate the new identity itself often leads eventually to the oblivion of death.)

The word "total" refers not simply to the comprehensive way in which the institution organizes all activities—eating, sleeping, working, leisure, and therapy sessions—but also to the strategies by which the institution invades the interior life of its inmates. In civilian life, Goffman observes, institutions usually claim the resident's overt behavior alone, releasing to the individual the question of his private attitude toward the organization. But in total institutions, the staff can legitimately busy itself with the resident's interior reactions to authority through a process that Goffman calls "looping." The resident finds to his dismay that his protective response to an assault upon his dignity itself collapses back into the situation and provides the staff with reasons for yet further controls; ". . . he cannot defend himself in the usual way by establishing distance between the mortifying situation and himself."[7] The all-monitoring eye of the supervisor surveys both his inner and his outer life and organizes the prison of his therapy.

THE MOTIVES FOR
INSTITUTIONALIZATION

However sensitively run, total institutions can exact from their residents a price, as they impose upon the segregated the ordeals of banishment and deprivation. What explanations can we offer for their attraction, above and beyond the original philanthropic impulses that founded them and the technical services they orchestrate? (I set aside in answer to this question the motives for entering the handsomely designed and expensive three-tier retirement centers to which the affluent elderly often move themselves.)

Philip Slater, a sociologist, offers the rawest explanation of their appeal in America. He argues that Americans are tempted to solve their problems by resorting to what he calls "the toilet assumption." We behave as though the most efficient and sanitary way of solving a problem is to avoid it by voiding it. To argue the depth of this tendency in the American character, Slater offered a revisionist view (in the *Pursuit of Loneliness*) on the motives of immigrants who settled this country. Our celebratory histories to the contrary, Americans were not the most heroic of Europe's millions. Rather, they were self-selectively those most inclined to solve the problems of an ancient continent and aging relatives by escaping from them. Americans have endlessly repeated this strategy of abandonment: as an immigrant people became a migratory people, moving from the East across the plains to the West; then, as a migratory people became a mobile people, leaving small towns in order to "make it" in the city; and then, after making our cities uninhabitable, fleeing from the city to the suburbs; and, finally, retreating from the tedium of the suburbs to the weekend retreat in the country. Slater sees in this ruthlessness the work of the toilet assumption—the American tendency to dispose of problems by flushing them.[8]

But why are we so drawn to the toilet assumption? Slater's attempt to explain it as a special character defect of those who migrated to America is historically dubious. Most immigrants did not come to the United States in order to flush the problems of their native countries. Certainly not the blacks, and probably not most of the whites. In his essay *Going to America*, Terry Colman notes that English absentee landlords in the late 1840s sought to get rid of huge numbers of Irish peasants on their estates by shipping them off to America. The practice was commonly known as "shoveling out."[9] It would appear that some of our forebears were not the flushers as much as the flushed.

Furthermore, if Michel Foucault's *Madness and Civilization* can be credited, Europeans in the Classical period of the seventeenth and eighteenth centuries already exhibited the tendency to solve problems by banishing a defiled population to a special institution. In this respect, the Age of Reason differed from the earlier medieval and renaissance worlds. Medieval society, according to Foucault, except for its treatment of lepers (and religious minorities), incarcerated its own members for reasons of deviancy much less often than did the reputedly more tolerant Age of Reason. Renaissance society let the mad and the indigent mingle in the society at large. But by the seventeenth and eighteenth centuries, rulers incarcerated the idle, the poor, the insane, and the criminal without distinction in lazar houses.

The religious ritual of confession, Foucault believes, helped shape and reflected the more generous, earlier medieval attitude toward deviancy. Confession concedes the fact of human imperfection, but also implies some confidence that evil can be let out into the open without engulfing those who pray. But classical Europe, with its proud celebration of human reason, "felt a shame in the presence of the inhuman"[10] that the earlier ages did not experience. After the seventeenth century, Western society increasingly assumed that one can handle evil only by banishing it. Put another way: an age that aspires to total autonomy admits with more difficulty the dependent, the defective, and the irrational into its life. These imperfect members of society represent a negativity so threatening and absolute that a society pretending to autonomy can only put them out of sight.

Foucault knew that this impulse to banish did not spring from a crude brutality. He recognized the philanthropic element in the move to sequester: "Interest in cure and expulsion coincide."[11] But it took David Rothman's *The Discovery of the Asylum* to show the intimate historical connection between the impulse to rehabilitate and the compulsion to segregate. The American historian documented the drastic change that occurred in the 1820s and afterward in the United States in the handling of crime, madness, and indigency. Until the early nineteenth century, Americans either whipped, pilloried, drove out of town, or hanged their criminals. Jails served as little more than temporary lockups until the penal system decided on the appropriate punishment. Not until the 1820s did this country adopt the strategy of building, and isolating criminals in, huge penitentiaries.

Similar changes occurred about the same time in the handling of the indigent and the insane. Until the 1820s, welfare funds largely supported families or surrogate families to take care of the poor. But increasingly in the nineteenth century, America constructed, and incarcerated the poor in, its great workhouses. Similarly, the country moved the mad from the attic and the hovel at the edge of town to the insane asylum.

Reformers made these changes for the philanthropic purpose of removing stricken populations from the evil influences of the society at large to the protected environment of the penitentiary or the asylum, where, under carefully controlled conditions (including isolation, work, discipline, and obedience under the authority of professionals), the distressed had a chance to recover. By the end of the Civil War, however, these massive, standardized facilities deteriorated into institutional bins, manned by professionals and subprofessional staff and filled with racial minorities.

In the medieval church, as a priest and his assistants dragged a leper out of the church with backward step and committed him to the lazar house, they would say to him: "And howsoever thou mayest be apart from the church and the company of the Sound, yet art thou not apart from the grace of God."[12] In the last one hundred years, our implied ritual address to the mad, the aged, and the criminal has been: "And howsoever thou mayest be apart from the community and the company of the Sound, yet art thou not apart from the ministrations of the Professional."

Thus rationalism, philanthropy, and professionalism intertwine with banishment and deprivation.

In my judgment, however, both Slater's attempt to locate the toilet assumption uniquely in the American immigrant experience and Foucault's effort to blame the impulse to banish exclusively on classical rationalism fail to persuade. Solving problems by dodging them dates back at least to the parable of the Good Samaritan. "Passing by on the other side" tempted ancient priests and levites as well as the modern middle class as a way of achieving some distance from the distressed. The impulses both to sequester and to devour spring from within humankind and not just idiosyncratically from careerist Americans or eighteenth-century rationalists.

We underestimate, moreover, the real power of these impulses within us in adopting too moralistic a view of their origin—in assuming that they issue from a gratuitous ruthlessness or complacency. Our neglect of the indigent does not result solely from the fact that we are too smug or too engrossed in our own riches to bother with them. If we examine our excuses for neglect,[13] including our reasons for institutionalization, we discover not so much smugness but anxiety, not self-assurance but a sense of harassment, not riches but a feeling of bankruptcy. The statement "I am too busy to care for her now" often betrays a free-floating anxiety: "I am riddled with concern about my own affairs. I can't break free from the grip of my own needs. They hold me in a vise. Maybe next year will be different. But this year is impossible."

Or again, the question "What can I do?" often blurts out no more than one's own despair: "I have nothing for the real needs of another because what I have doesn't satisfy my own. What help could I possibly offer him? It is better to avoid him. To face him would be too depressing. He would remind me of the emptiness of my own fate." Many a man avoids a visit to the bed of a dying friend for reason of the latter dread.

He knows he has nothing to say that will help. He feels resourceless before his friend's imminent death and his own. He himself is in need, and a face-to-face meeting with his friend would remind him of his own exigency.

Not all expediency in our treatment of the distressed springs from gross callousness; rather, we are busily engaged in obscuring from view our own poverty: both hiding from ourselves and hiding our selves. We consign to oblivion the maimed, the disfigured, and the decrepit, because we have already condemned to oblivion a portion of ourselves. To address them in their needs would require us to permit ourselves to be addressed in our needs. But we recoil from accepting the depths of our own neediness. The hidden away threaten us with what we have already hidden away from ourselves. For some such reason, we prefer, even at great expense, to remove them from sight. And what better way to place them in the shadows and to obscure our own neediness, than to hand them over to professionals whose métier it is to make a show of strength, experience, and competence in handling a given subdivision of the distressed? Thus the exigent provide an opportunity for the community to exhibit its precedence and power over them.

A CONCLUDING COMMENT

Three major and differing political reactions have emerged in interpreting the problems raised in this essay—conservative, reformist, and revolutionary. These reactions require comment in the light of the religious tradition that engages me as a theologian.

The modern, pragmatic, libertarian conservative would find in David Rothman's account of the emergence and decline of the asylum vindication for his skepticism about reform. The degeneration of the asylum provides but another sad tale of reform gone to seed. In the brief period of forty years, institutions with utopian aspirations deteriorated into dumping grounds for the desperate. Why bother, Mr. Reformer? Spare me your plans and save me some change.

Hobbes and his latter-day descendants among conservatives would darken this particular historical lesson into a comprehensive pessimism. Our institutions can do little more than keep human misery in check because of the murderous appetites to which human beings are subject. The impulses to sequester and devour derive from human nature; they are not just a cultural accident. Hobbes provided the anthropological foundations for this claim by observing: animals hunger only with the hunger of the moment, but man, like Satan, hungers and thirsts *infinitely*. His boundless, devouring hunger makes man "the most predatory, the most cunning, the strongest, and the most dangerous animal."[14] Moreover, Hobbes linked, by implication, this activity of devouring with the further impulse to sequester when he argued that men characteristically differ from animals in their "striving after honor and positions of honor, after precedence over others and recognition of this precedence by others, ambition, pride, and the passion for fame."[15] One man's glory demands another man's eclipse. When we aspire to step forward into the light, we betray the underside of this aspiration in our readiness to see others overshadowed by our illumination. Man's boundless craving, and specifically his appetite for honor and precedence, generates that enmity among humankind which justifies, in Hobbes's estimate, his characterization of the state of nature as "solitary, poor, nasty, brutish, and short." Thus, devouring and overshadowing connect, and our fears that others will devour and surpass us reinforce these murderous impulses. Hobbes resolved our sorry plight by arguing that we must accept our irrevocable duties of obedience to the state and its agencies, which, albeit oppressive, exercise a monopoly over the power of death and thereby keep terror within limits.

In their differing ways, both conservative skepticism and Hobbesian pessimism justify the *status quo* or the *status quo ante* for those institutions that consume, consign to oblivion, or oppress. Hobbes warns, in effect, leave well enough alone. Things are bad, but could be worse. Neither the skeptic nor the Hobbesian conservative appreciates the very real differences institutions (and public institutions) can make, not just in maintaining order, but in aspiring to the good. Without some sense of the distinctions between better and worse and the ineliminable and the reformable, one leaves very little room for improving the lot of the needy, ourselves included.

At the opposite end of the political spectrum, utopian reformers and revolutionaries tend to locate death in our institutional life alone. They see individuals and groups as relatively innocent victims of an oppressive social order. The reformer does battle with social evils, discrete and episodic, in the hope of making things better. But the revolutionary views the specter of overtaxed clinics in ghetto neighborhoods, rotting vegetables in wards, infected blood in banks, and foul overcrowding in jails as symptoms of a generally discredited social and political structure. The system serves the excellors and the devourers rather than the failed and the deprived. Since, however, individuals and groups are relatively innocent victims of the system, reformers and revolutionaries believe that humankind possesses the moral resources either for the piecemeal improvement of the system (the reformer's aim) or for the total displacement of the current system by one superior to it (the revolutionary's hope).

The positions of Hobbesian conservatives and of revolutionaries, like many other opposites, ultimately resemble one another. Both parties think too globally. The conservative wholly justifies and the revolutionary wholly repudiates institutions as they are. As such, they fail to distinguish sufficiently between varied total institutions, better and worse, and to discriminate among varied proposals for their discrete improvement. The chapters in this volume on the institutionalized retarded and on the aged attempt to show some of those qualities of total institutions that make them both indispensable and praiseworthy and the workers and residents within them deserving of our admiration. Thus, while I have emphasized in this chapter the ordeals which institutionalization imposes, I have not done so with the intent of repudiating the institutions. They impose some ordeals intrinsically and inevitably and others gratuitously. Wise reforms will eliminate the gratuitous, reduce to a minimum the inevitable, improve the necessary, and reserve institutionalization to as small a population as possible.

What response can one make theologically to these contending general assessments of institutions in our time? Reinhold Niebuhr offered the most influential theological response during the period under review. Niebuhr faulted the Hobbesian pessimists for locating destructiveness exclusively within the murderous impulses of humankind and for dealing too kindly with its institutional manifestations. However, Niebuhr also criticized the reformers and the revolutionary optimists for locating oppression exclusively in the social system and for exculpating individuals and groups as its relatively innocent victims. Niebuhr urged, instead, a more complex anthropology that sought to do justice both to the human and institutional capacity for good and to the individual and social capacity for destructiveness.

While salutary, Niebuhr's theological response did not address the more metaphysical question that underlies the social debates of our time. Both parties to the political debate, despite their differences, share in common a somewhat gloomy metaphysical vision. They both tend to define their politics by the experience of death and destruction alone. Conservatives justify institutions and revolutionaries justify their overthrowal in reaction to a negativity rather than to the experience of some positive, nurturant power which may offer hope of rebirth and thus authorizes their action. The fear of death and destruction keeps the conservative defensive about institutions; the hatred of death often provokes the revolutionary to attack them.

Fear supplies the hydraulic fluid and pressure that make the system work for the Hobbesian conservative. Inasmuch as institutions derive their power from the fear of death, we cannot expect them to dispense with this fear. Leviathan—and all its attendant institutions—deserves a monopoly over the power of death for fear of that even more murderous state of affairs that afflicts us in a state of nature without its ministrations.

Correspondingly, the hatred of death usually provides revolutionaries and often reformers with their life's meaning and vocation. Such activists may rightly see the evils of the system, but wrongly define their vocation by that perception alone. Evil serves them as that absolute which authorizes their activities and shapes their plans for a new or better society. They seek relentlessly to eliminate the negative from human life as their passion and calling.

Perhaps the eighteenth century European and nineteenth century American experiments with total institutions teach a somewhat different lesson. They emphasize that an ethic defined by resistance alone usually imposes on others what it seeks to depose. The total institution failed partly because it operated reflexively against negativities, the absolute negativities of madness, crime, dependency, and decrepitude. Society assumed that the negative absolutely must be eliminated (through the ministrations of the professional) and, when it cannot be eliminated, it must be sequestered or eliminated by being sequestered.

It may be less pernicious to assume that the negative is not absolute and therefore that its elimination is not the precondition of a truly human existence. Once conservatives, reformers, and revolutionaries no longer treat negativities as absolutes, then the conservative may be less tempted to justify institutional repression and reformers less tempted to lay upon professionals the fatal charge to eliminate negativity or to banish ruthlessly its host. This deflation of evil, moreover, need not lead to quietism or complacency. Action against evil does not require that we inflate it absolutely.

Where, however, does one find theological warrant for this alternative vision of the metaphysical setting in which social action takes place? In my own efforts to puzzle over this problem as a Christian theologian, I have found myself drawn to the passages about the "suffering servant" in Isaiah. Remarkably enough, the text locates God's servant in the very arena of death that we have been exploring. He exposed himself to deprivation and oblivion. "He was despised and rejected by men; a man of sorrows and acquainted with grief, and as one from whom men hide their faces, he was despised, and we esteemed him not" (Isaiah 53:3).

The passage furthermore does not suggest that this move into the site of deprivation and death engulfs him. Though "he was cut off from the land of the living" and though he "poured out his soul to death," his resources do not thereby deplete or thin out. Quite the contrary: in and through his outpouring of service, the will of the Lord actually prospers in his hand. God's servant "suffers"—not simply as tortured, but as determinedly subject to the will of God. God may will him to places where he must endure. But his suffering resembles more "suffer the little children to come unto me" than "look what suffering I have endured for your sake, ungrateful woman!" He suffers but also suffers as an attending to, a following, a tracking after the powerful will that creates, preserves, and upholds in love. Therefore, the passage suggests a peculiarly intimate connection between love's flourishing and his own dying.[16]

The assertion of any such link between dying and prospering contrasts starkly with our ordinary conception of social action. In traditional social action, we assume some kind of dualistic battle in which either we gradually prevail over death (in which case death diminishes) or we find our resources gradually thinned out by death (in which case we diminish). But this passage suggests that the suffering servant makes his own dying, that is, his own laying down of his life, an essential ingredient in that life which he shares with the community. "By his stripes we are healed."

Christians have traditionally drawn a moral implication from this passage. A community that professes such a servant as savior cannot avoid going into places marked by rejection, pain, and oblivion. In failing to do so, the community would defect from its own mission in the God from whom no secret places are hid.

Concretely, such a savior demands of the churches that they not leave health care exclusively in the hands of the bureaucracies and their professional staffs which serve as the current chief instruments of a society's sequestering. The churches must find ways to open themselves up to loving the institutionalized needy: (1) to provide supplemental services above and beyond those that the bureaucracies can provide; (2) to criticize bureaucracies for their failure to provide what they ought to provide and thereby to assist in their improvement; (3) to encourage the development of alternative delivery systems where appropriate; and (4) to provide the community at large with sufficient contact with the plight of the deprived and the forlorn so as to effect a more favorable ethos in the society toward them and the ordeals that beset them.

But a moralistic reading of the passage from Isaiah does not cut through to the nerve of the problem. The problem we face consists not simply of other people's suffering but of our own. We avoid the failures of others because we cannot bear to see our own failures reflected in their faces; we deprive the needy because we absorbingly attempt to overcome our own limitless sense of deprivation; and rarely are we so tempted to impose pain on others as when we are hellbent on relieving it, convinced of the absolute righteousness of our cause and the indispensability of our contribution in promoting that cause.

Thus the final word spoken in Isaiah 53 must address our own metaphysical plight.

If the anointed of God has exposed himself to deprivation and oblivion, then men and women need fear no longer that the death and failure that they know in themselves can separate them from God. Those powers they fear as absolute have been rendered of no account, either as they appear in them or as they beset their fellow creatures.

This position of metaphysical optimism differs from the vision of the conservative who elevates the powers of darkness and disorder into a divine figure of chaos which institutions must grimly contain; and it differs from the pessimism of the revolutionary whose cause derives its inspiration from the repressive institutional negativity that he seeks to overcome. The act of dying for others penetrates, rather than sidesteps or merely reacts to, the negative. Death looms as one of the principalities and powers, to be sure, but a creature for all of that, incapable of separating human beings from the substance of self-expending love. As this love takes hold of men and women, they suffer rebirth, perhaps in blood and fire, perhaps in water, but, in any event, reconnected to creative, nurturant, and donative love.

This vision of the human plight should not undercut the motive for works of mercy and relief among people and the reformation of defective institutions. Quite the contrary, it should enable them, for it deprives the negative of its ultimacy and therefore its power to paralyze, dominate, and distort. It relieves men and women of the burden of messianism. They need no longer repress the negative in themselves, or impose it on others, or obsess on it in their enemies, or protect themselves from it through the shield of the professional. They can freely perform whatever acts of kindness they can and even receive such acts from others, as a limited sign of a huge mercy which their own works have not produced.

THE AFFLICTED
ASSISTING
THE AFFLICTED
Alcoholics Anonymous

USUALLY THE AFFLICTED seek help from a fee-charging expert. But the AA movement began when a struggling alcoholic stockbroker on a business trip in Akron, Ohio approached a local physician for his personal experience, not his professional expertise: the physician himself suffered from alcoholism. After telling his story, the stockbroker confessed, "I called Henrietta [the go-between] because I needed another alcoholic. I needed you, Bob, probably more than you'll ever need me. So thanks a lot for hearing me out. I know now that I'm not going to take a drink, and I'm grateful to you."[1] Dr. Bob, in response, offered his own story. The exchange established a to and fro, in which an afflicted assisted another afflicted who assisted, in turn, the assisting afflicted. The date shortly thereafter on which Dr. Bob took his last drink in Atlantic City —June 10, 1935—marks the official birthday of Alcoholics Anonymous.[2]

The emergence of AA in 1935 spotlights a little-noticed irony in modern medicine. On the one hand, health care practice has relentlessly professionalized in the twentieth century. The transfer of professional training from the apprenticeship system into the universities both symbolized and furthered this process. This shift declared that effective therapy springs from a complex and esoteric body of knowledge wholly inaccessible to the lay person. Patients consume health care; they cannot provide it. Research in the university, the development of specialties, and the multiplication of subspecialties underline the message that healing depends upon occult knowledge wholly hidden from the lay person.

The afflicted, this message continues, benefit from the ministrations of complexly trained professionals, but they can neither help nor safely accept help from one another. As the saying goes, a little knowledge is a dangerous thing.

Yet, during the same time that the experts, whom the universities had created and ordained, seized control of health care, lay communities of care have burgeoned, proliferated, and subdivided into specialized groups offering mutual help and support. The boundary lines between these support groups often reflect the boundaries between the professional specializations: the burned, the addicted, MS patients, heart attack victims, diabetics, cancer patients of various types, the multiply-handicapped, paraplegics, the battered, the molested, and the obese form groups that offer mutual lay help. Further, the families of those patients who cannot help themselves have also organized, such as the parents of prematures or the families of the retarded, the mentally ill, or the senile. As the primary, daily caregivers for those with massive needs, families themselves qualify as afflicted. Whatever the ordeal, a specialized community has organized itself to assist those who have more recently suffered it, and thereby also, according to testimony, they have helped themselves.

One of the twenty-seven clearinghouses for mutual support groups in the USA puts out a directory, *The Self-Help Sourcebook*, that lists the other twenty-six clearinghouses and over 525 national self-help groups.[3] A *New York Times* article, July 16, 1988, estimates that 12 to 15 million people in North America belong to some 500,000 self-help organizations (including local chapters).[4] Some of these organizations have flickered in and out of existence like fireflies. Others date back to the 1930s and 1940s and have thrown lifelines to their members for fifty years or more. Some specialized support groups offer help to each of the afflicted covered in this volume: the burned (The Phoenix Society, the National Burn Victim Foundation); the battered (Batterers Anonymous and many diverse local shelters for battered women); the abused (Incest Survivors Anonymous, Sexual Assault Recovery Anonymous Society, Parents United); the aged (four groups, including the Gray Panthers and the American Association of Retired Persons); the retarded (seven groups, including support groups for the parents and siblings of the retarded).

The growth of these lay communities of support alongside the professional organizations of specialists should not surprise us. The very success of modern medicine has imposed upon patients and their families extraordinary burdens of rehabilitative and chronic care, burdens which previously they would not have had to carry. Today families often must bear the new burden of extended care before they endure the customary suffering of bereavement. Further, the increased mobility and transiency of people in the modern world has broken down traditional social support systems. We can no longer rely on aunts, uncles, cousins, or even adult brothers and sisters and must perforce appeal to an extended community of fellow sufferers, a community which affliction, not blood, has defined.

Alcoholics Anonymous showed the way for many self-help groups organized since the mid-1930s by victims to help fellow victims. Dr. Bob and stockbroker Bill, with their mutually shared life stories of repeated defeat and despair and their final resort to higher power, started AA in the little churches of healing which they and their colleagues and spiritual descendants have established in this country and abroad. Alcoholics Anonymous generated Al Anon (for relatives and friends of drinkers), Alateen (for children of alcoholics still in the household or young enough to be in the household), even Alatot, and, most recently, COA (the adult Children of Alcoholics, an organization which, like the others, has grown rapidly and remains loosely organized). AA also provided a model for many of the other self-help groups formed by victims to assist other victims to face the catastrophes which threaten to overwhelm and which, if survived, often require the survivor to alter identity. It influenced especially groups formed to deal with particular addictions, but also, in part, other groups organized to cope with diseases or with stressful life circumstances. The discussion in this chapter, while confined to AA, closes with some of the similarities and differences that other types of mutual support groups display.

Alcoholics Anonymous combines the two ways of looking at moral problems with which this book began. AA emphasizes, on the one hand, the ethics of problem-solving. Nothing could be more catechetical and casuistical than the AA literature and rituals as they specify the steps the victim must take to resolve a problem that besets and often overwhelms some twelve to fifteen million Americans and lacerates and scars their spouses, children, and companions. AA literature fairly bristles with slogans and advice and practical comments: "first things first," "one day at a time," "easy does it," "live and let live," "I am responsible," "go to meetings," "keep it simple," "progress rather than perfection," "the first drink gets the alcoholic drunk," "you can do something but not everything," "don't promise never to drink again, rather, don't take the first drink—one day at a time," "keep coming back," "it works," "everyone is equal here." The movement helps the alcoholic go from "I cannot drink" to "I can not-drink." These slogans fit into the kind of problem-solving advice that authors turn out endlessly for the readers of "do-it-yourself" literature.

And yet, the AA movement breaks with this conventional, problem-solving, do-it-yourself ethics in two ways. First, strictly speaking, AA does not claim that alcoholics (or therapists) can solve their problem. As the slogan puts it, you never get over being an alcoholic. The problem sticks, it endures. It is a hardy perennial: it will always sprout again.

The alcoholic stays an alcoholic until he dies. The alcoholic who thinks he can solve the problem once and for all cannot solve it at all. Further, the key problem requires not the resolution of a quandary but the redefinition of the alcoholic's own self. Therefore, AA deals not with tidy cases but with rambling stories. Significantly, "The Book" (*Alcoholics Anonymous*), the basic AA volume, published in 1939 and reprinted in several editions, begins with a chapter entitled "Bill's Story" and devotes over two-thirds of the remainder to another forty-three stories. Ethics, in this setting, does not solve casuistically but recitatively. If the Twelve Steps supply the movement with its law, the personal narratives supply the movement with its shaping stories; those stories encourage, inspire, and enable sufferers to follow the path which the Twelve Steps blaze.[5] The AA meetings similarly help members to internalize the law—the Twelve Steps—by sharing members' stories.

In effect, the movement begins with two people talking and listening to one another. The alcoholic is awash in his own life-long monologue; he needs dialogue. No one can break through to dialogue on his own; nor does he participate in it by listening to an onslaught of sermons and warnings from others. Dialogue takes two. "There could not have been just one founder of AA. There had to be two, because the essence of the process is one person telling his story to another as honestly as he knows how."[6]

Exchanging stories establishes a community. That community differs from the others the world conventionally prizes: men and women gather together not on the basis of what they possess—race, religion, intelligence, property, money, achievement, education, or class identity—but on the basis of what they lack. This community derives not from possession, but from need. It offers "a sharing union with others in a mutual acceptance rooted in weakness rather than strength."[7] Whatever change—spiritual or otherwise—the alcoholic undergoes by participating in this community, he cannot think of this alteration as an acquisition. For the alteration itself grows from acknowledged need, primordial, chronic, and continuing. In this need or lack lies the common ground the religious and the nonreligious members of AA share. "Within Alcoholics Anonymous, the promise of anonymity made possible the acceptance of oneself as limited. Sharing this acceptance with others who were similarly limited . . . in turn made possible acceptance of self as not-God, as men and women made whole by the acceptance of limitation."[8]

The stories members tell follow a pattern. The image of death and rebirth shows up in the alcoholic's story, just as surely as in the Dax story with which this volume began. The wife of an alcoholic said, ". . . all these people would be dead if it weren't for each other."[9] One hears constantly from the beginner, "I am dying," or from the veteran, recounting his story, "I was dying."[10] Such comments remind one of the Gerasene demoniac in the New Testament who "lived among the tombs" (Mark 5:3). Emphasizing rebirth, Nan Robertson reports that leaders of meetings often ask, "Is anybody celebrating a birthday this week?"[11] To which question, at one meeting, a "young man with a black pirate's mustache shoots up his hand . . . smiles sheepishly and says, 'My name is Len, and I'm an alcoholic, and I'm two years in AA next Monday.' Everyone claps; the man next to Len puts an arm over his shoulders and says, 'Way to go!' "[12] The alcoholic organizes his calendar from that date marking his first meeting. "The newer a person is, the more enthusiastic the clapping, because all members know that the first days and weeks without a drink are the hardest."[13] Just as the members organize their new lives and calendar from the day they entered the program, so the movement organizes its calendar from its birthdate, the day when the second of the co-founders, Dr. Bob, took his last drink (June 10, 1935). The institutional birthdate makes possible the personal dates of birth. "I was dying and the program gave me hope."[14]

The pseudonymous author of the memoir "A Drunkard's Progress," published in Harper's in 1986,[15] compares the alcoholic's story to a fairytale. Like most fairytales, it includes a quest and an ordeal. Telling his tale helps heal the storyteller and the listener. Drunk, the alcoholic creates possible selves, fantastical selves. Telling his story, the alcoholic recollects and remembers those selves, and thereby can return to himself, sober up. He moves from lies to reality—the pilgrim's progress in both the fairytale and the religious pilgrimage. Freudians classify the alcoholic as oral/infantile in personality.[16] He sucks the bottle. He seeks destruction through his lips, and perforce he must recover by changing the way he uses his lips by telling his story. He must move from the baby's fixation on the oral to an adult's. He must move from spirits to the spiritual through the sharing of stories that allows for the self's own recovery. Once again the language reminds one of the religious traditions of healing. Healing the Gerasene demoniac restores him to "his right mind" (Mark 5:15).

Some interpreters refuse to recognize this story pattern as religious. They have noted that the AA Preamble, read at many AA meetings, distances itself from official religious institutions: "AA is not allied with any sect, denomination, politics, organization, or institution. . . ." AA also balks at the homiletical, evangelical tendencies of Protestant Christianity and the absolutism of the Oxford Movement, whose chain of informal, intimate prayer groups admittedly influenced the AA founders. The AA winces at "preaching," which, as I have said, violates the possibility of equal sharing. Hectoring alcoholics with the Oxford Movement's four absolutes would only face them with their own inevitable failure and confirm their sense of their own flaws. Nan Robertson concedes that pious, churchy language crops up in AA meetings outside her home base in New York City, but she considers the "God part" detachable and dispensable.[17] She and others note that the movement has always described itself as "spiritual" rather than "religious."

In preferring the term "spiritual," the AA movement clearly tries to distinguish itself from conventional, organized religious bodies and their theologies. While some of the Twelve Steps refer to God, none reflects an interest in theological questions about God's nature. Rather, the Steps explicitly defer to each alcoholic's own personal sense of God —"as he [or she] understands Him." At first glance, this theological indifferentism seems to follow tactically from the mission of AA. Attempting to reach out to all alcoholics, the organization rejects any definition or God-language that might scare off any in need, whatever their creed—Jews, Roman Catholics, Lutherans, Pentecostals, Eastern Orthodox communicants, Buddhists, humanists, or secularists.

This theological reserve, however, rests on a second consideration, more substantive than tactical. Both the language of the Twelve Steps and the autobiographical statements of alcoholics reflect a fairly instinctive but apt sense of the essence of religion as it illuminates the struggle which each alcoholic faces. The term "religion," as used in the Twelve Steps, refers to a personal and passionate experience of power rather than to the conventional theological formulas promulgated by various denominations. The Twelve Steps reflect "religion" as meaning "Power," not "institution." The "religious" and the "spiritual" intersect in the word "power," a word which provides the key to the alcoholic's biography. "Power," appears, capitalized, twenty times in the chapter on "We Agnostics" in *Alcoholics Anonymous*[18] and several times in the Twelve Steps. The term stamps the movement as inescapably religious in its spirituality. The alcoholic affirms "Step One: We admitted that we were *powerless* over alcohol in our past—that our lives had become unmanageable; Step Two: [we] came to believe that *power* greater than ourselves could restore us to sanity; Step Three: [we] made a decision to turn our will and our lives over to the care of God as we understood Him; . . . Step Eleven: [we] sought through prayer and meditation to improve conscious contact with God as we understood Him, praying only for knowledge of His will for us and the *power* to carry that out."[19]

Religion at its deepest levels has always emphasized access to "Power," as does the AA. The phenomenologists of religion say that "religion" does not originally center on a deity. The "gods," argues Van der Leeuw,[20] arrived relatively late on the scene in the history of religion. Long before the gods appeared, religion consisted of some sort of experience of sacred or supernatural power, a *"tremendum,"* alien and overpowering and yet alluring. However it shows itself, the supernatural differs from profane power; it does not allow men and women to master and control it and use it for their own ends. It insists upon unfolding in its own way, on disrupting the procedures by which people ordinarily handle their lives.

At the outset, of course, liquor does not appear to offer too bad a bargain. It partly overpowers through its allure. The *tremendum* appears as a *"fascinosum"*; it overwhelms partly through its fascination. Liquor offers some pleasure; it bolsters confidence; it encourages candor among friends and intimacy with a lover. It inspirits a gathering and secures release from a bad day. But, above all else, it expands the alcoholic's sense of power. It lets him feel he can command the demon that W. H. Auden once called "Possibility," the same demon the gambler wants to command. The pseudonymous "Elpenor" writes in *Harper's*, "We drank to spawn new selves, to be reborn in Possibility, more charming, more persuasive, more resolute, more high-spirited. . . ." Possibility appears as "the achingly elusive element in which we live and move and have our dreams, the drowning pool of the self."[21] As the self inflates and expands, alcohol lets Faust believe he can make himself emperor, magician, scientist, novelist, ranking salesman, and sexually and socially adept. It lures him giddily beyond his actual self, which seems so lacking by comparison in luster and self-confidence. Thus even as the self inflates and expands, the alcoholic rebels against being himself and rebels against the authorities in his life—his mother, his father, his wife (now mother)—but subtly, in a form that still defines him as weak, dependent, and therefore in need of their continuing care.

Meanwhile, the roistering *bonhomie* that liquor engenders temporarily suspends for the alcoholic a sense of his own social mistakes so that his shortcomings appear less hopeless. Liquor temporarily short-circuits the moral computer within—the bookkeeper who adds up guilt and the registrar who records shame. Admittedly, this side of oblivion the drinker may notice that booze leads him to foolish actions and dangerous moods. It keys up his anger and seems to justify his verbal, physical, and even sexual violence. It marinates him in self-pity and makes him a boring companion, as he endlessly reruns his grievances and sounds the same plaintive tones again and again, like an idiot violinist who bows his favorite notes over and over. But, even while the alcoholic takes marginal note of all this, he feels that he himself has not lost control; his core self remains untouched; he could, if he wanted to, reassert himself and master his problem.

This self-deception forms a substantial part of liquor's power. The alcoholic tells himself that he needs only to make up his mind to limit himself to a shot in the morning or only two martinis at lunch, or wait for the sun to set, or switch from hard liquor to wine, or drink only when others are around, or only on the weekends when it does not matter. All these comforting stories mislead to the degree that they masquerade as options. Alcohol seems a mere additive to life, something that he can pour in or not at will, assimilate into his life as part of a whole, like the other powers that he manages, manipulates, and controls.

Step One in the Twelve Steps bluntly rejects this picture of his plight. The alcoholic publicly acknowledges that he is "powerless over alcohol."[22] Powerlessness characterizes his true condition. Indeed, his power has so failed that he abjectly serves the enemy that is destroying him. His reason, most of all, serves his addiction, first in the form of denial, and then by going over to the enemy, as it were, and humbly aiding and abetting his addiction. Reason helps him invent the lies he tells himself about his control over booze and then helps him invent excuses for believing those lies. It furnishes a hundred ingenious excuses as to why he needs a drink, a second, or a third. It humbly serves as supply officer, arranging for a steady flow of the material that will destroy him. It dutifully figures out the logistics of how to store liquor in appropriate locations and camouflage it to prevent its interception and confiscation. It helps him administer enough of it to himself, over a life-long period of siege, so as to annihilate himself. Suicide by inches, or "chronic suicide," Karl Menninger once called alcohohlism.[23]

At length, the alcoholic finds himself gripped by a power that renders him powerless. This power acts like a vengeful and malicious god, not a creative, nurturant, and preservative deity. The alcoholic experiences power as dominating and abusive. Eventually it wholly owns him and threatens to destroy him and those he loves. He experiences the sacred as demonic, a word trivialized in our time to suggest fire-breathing, horned, cloven-hoofed, and semicomic figures. The alcoholic, however, experiences the demonic as wholly destructive power. Liquor thickens the tongue, bloats the liver, dehydrates and emaciates the body, wipes out reaches of memory, impairs judgment, damages the brain, blackens moods, jangles nerves, routs the wife, shames the children, drives away friends, ruins the work record, and reduces the alcoholic to total despair. In the end, alcohol enforces the only rhythm left in his life: drink, hangover, and drink again.

The ruthless honesty of Step One, while necessary, does not suffice. It would simply arouse in the alcoholic an abject fear of his own weakness against liquor's destructive power. As a former drug addict testified, fear alone never persuaded a single alcoholic to give up the bottle. The alcoholic needs to take a second step, a step toward a power that surpasses his own and the power of alcohol. Only such a power can help him radically reorient his life.

This reorientation does not eliminate his weakness and dependency; he stops depending on liquor and authority figures, and begins to trust an utterly transcendent power. This transcendent power (the Book calls it, variously, "Creative Intelligence," "a Spirit of the Universe," "the Realm of the Spirit . . . broad, roomy, all inclusive")[24] redefines the alcoholic. He need no longer assume that his own violent mood swings will govern his actions. He can instead believe that an encompassing and stable power will let him totally surrender and reconstitute his life. The handbook states it bluntly: "Lack of power, that was our dilemma. We had to find a power by which we could live, and it had to be a Power greater than ourselves,"[25] greater not only than the power of alcohol, but greater than all *human* power—the alcoholic's, the parents', the spouse's, and the doctor's included.[26]

Thus alcoholics reach the "decision," in Step Three, "to turn our lives over to the care of God as we understood him."[27] Surrendering one's willfulness and self-assertion requires powerful and alien help from beyond. This surrender differs from submitting to doctors and clinics, which only superficially modify behavior. The merely compliant alcoholic may accept the physician's regimen, but he does so tentatively, experimentally, always ready to change his mind, to accept the unexpected free drink from a friend, or to assent to a skeptical turn of phrase from a companion. In Step Three, however, the self must enlist for the duration, rather than decide to drill from time to time.

Sometimes self-assertion lurks beneath an apparently comprehensive surrender; the self congratulates itself, saying, "As opposed to others who partially comply, I have wholly surrendered myself." That soul surrenders because it decides to surrender; such a surrender still relies upon the self's own resolution. And what the self has done, it can undo. True surrender, on the other hand, requires the self to cast itself upon a Power that surpasses its own treacherous powers, the awesome and proven power of alcohol, and the limited powers of the medical professional.

Put traditionally, the self must undergo a radical conversion, and comprehensively reorient. It must learn to take on, accept, and let grow within itself a new dependency, an absolute dependency upon transcendent power. Dr. Harry M. Tiebout has explored the psychological complexity of this total surrender, and its liberating dependency.[28] Dependency does not liberate absolutely since the alcoholic can never truthfully say that he is no longer an alcoholic. He can never relegate his alcoholism to the past tense. And yet, transcendent power has empowered him. He has moved from a resentful perception of his weakness —"I cannot drink (like other people)"—to a perception of a new power: "I can not-drink."[29] This empowerment he must reacquire daily through liberating prayer and meditation (Steps Six, Seven, and Eleven): he must reorder his relation not only to God but also to his neighbor and to himself (Steps Four, Five, and Eight).

In addition to alcohol's physical and social destructiveness—its damage to the body and the brain, to work and marriage—the alcoholic must recognize its spiritual destructiveness, the burdens of guilt and shame which the alcoholic bears and which often raise an almost insuperable obstacle to recovery. The alcoholic experiences the dead weight of both guilt and shame; and conversion and recovery must deal with both. The line between guilt and shame, according to Ernest Kuntz, shows up in two kinds of self-reproaches. Guilt accuses: "How could I have done *that!*" Shame reproaches: "How could *I* have done that!"[30]

Guilt springs from discrete, specific acts of commission and omission whereby the alcoholic has harmed others. Thus Step Four requires alcoholics to make a "searching and fearless moral inventory" of themselves. The "inventory" requires a list of discrete deeds and specific harms. The required "fearlessness" cuts through the rationalizations that flow from fear. Previously the alcoholic drowns his knowledge of what he has done in liquor. Otherwise, the injuries and wrongs he committed and the duties he dodged would spook and haunt him. Fear helped drive him to the bottle, to lying to himself and others. But, surrendering to Power, he can now make his moral inventory contritely without fearing that he will simply drive himself deeper into the pain of remorse.

The theological tradition carefully distinguishes between remorse and contrition. It calls remorse "earthly sorrow" because remorse merely heaps painful memories upon the original pain of the act. Remorse literally means biting again. The remorseful lie awake at bedtime, reliving the injuries they committed earlier in the day and reopening their own wounds. Remorse leads to a dead end. It rejects the future; it locks one in the boxes of the past and present. Surrender, however, opens contrition to the alcoholic. The "godly sorrow" of contrition, that is, sorrow from the vantage point of the transcendent Power, opens the future to the repentant. It makes possible confession (Step Five) and steps toward reparation (Steps Eight and Nine).

Step Five requires, however, that alcoholics not exaggerate the injuries they have inflicted on others. It requires that we admit "to God, to ourselves, and to another human being the *exact* nature of our wrongs," no more and no less. The alcoholic inclines to what Thomas Aquinas called the sins of defect and excess with respect to the truth: either reluctance to admit the real harm, or an exaggerated self-disparagement that covertly magnifies the dramatic importance of the self. AA's autobiographical vignettes amply demonstrate the alcoholic's propensity to the pretension that theology calls the sin of singularity —not, in this case, the pretension to a theatrical uniqueness in virtue, but in vice. The alcoholic tends to exaggerate his failings just as theatrically as the grandiose puff up their spiritual triumphs. The required exactness of Step Five provides the antidote to the alcoholic's narcissistic preoccupation with the self—whether exalted or abased beyond its due.

Specific acts of reparation provide important steps through the door into the future which moral inventories and contrition have opened. Steps Eight and Nine recommend listing all persons harmed and making "direct amends to such people, whenever possible, except when to do so would injure them or others." The last advisory recognizes that in the barbed tangle of human affairs some confessions of wrongdoing and efforts at amends would only injure some parties afresh. Marital infidelity offers an example. While confession might satisfy the alcoholic's sense of moral fastidiousness and drama, his "clean breast of it" might exact a heavy price from his spouse and succeed only in further humiliating and hurting her. The Twelve Steps keep the alcoholic from throwing not only confessions but reparations into the whirlpool of narcissism.

The alcoholic's problem goes deeper than guilt—it sinks into shame. In Kurtz's typology, guilt springs from doing wrong, but shame from being flawed; guilt from a sense of wickedness, shame from a sense of worthlessness; guilt from causing pain, shame from feeling pain; guilt from the wrong exercise of power and control, shame from the lack of power and control; guilt from the not-good, shame from the no-good; guilt from injuring others, and shame from demeaning the self. Guilt is objective; shame is subjective.

Shame is profoundly self-referential, so much so that whereas we speak of the opposite of guilt as guiltless, we do not call the opposite of shame shameless. Whereas the ashamed perceives his self as worthless, the shameless has lost a sense of worth (and of self) and therefore of the worth or worthlessness of the self.[31] Shame afflicts and therefore ultimately posits a core identity. Shame does not spring simply from the deeds of an agent, but rather from those deeds as they reflect backward into one's core being or lack thereof. Hollow men cannot feel shame.

(At one point Kurtz equates his distinction between guilt and shame with the traditional existentialist distinction between moral guilt and existential guilt. Moral guilt, according to the existentialists, refers to discrete deeds through which one person violates or neglects another. The existentialist's notion of existential guilt roughly corresponds to Kurtz's notion of shame; it springs from that deep fault or crack within one's being that transcends all specific actions. This existential guilt springs from existence as such; it fosters our sense that we have been thrown into an alien and hostile existence rather than born and bonded into community, that one survives and endures altogether outside of community, never within it. This perceived alienation assuredly resembles the ache of being which the alcoholic, but not the alcoholic alone, feels.

But this existentialist perception of a fault and lack in being also differs from the alcoholic's perception: first, the alcoholic perceives the fault in his being as a lack of goodness; second, AA does not enjoy the existentialist's confidence that one can withstand this lack by taking it upon oneself. The AA movement believes that the alcoholic's feeling of lack and weakness can ease only as he recognizes that he is not God, that he has not, in and of himself, the fullness and plenitude of supreme being; he thus must freely open to transcendent Power and reconnect with that special community that so openly and unashamedly acknowledges its profound and reflexive experience of itself as flawed.)

Guilt springs from deeds, but shame from the deeper issue of identity. Thus Steps Six and Seven abandon the language of discrete acts of reparation and suggest the language of reconnected or "born again" identity—"Ready to have God remove all these defects of character" and "humbly asked Him to remove our shortcomings." This reconnecting treats God as Polestar; hence, Step Eleven seeks "through prayer and meditation to improve our conscious contact with God." But this reconnecting also points the initiate to the inner community of Alcoholics Anonymous, that is, to other, similar, flawed, desperate, powerless, human individuals who have joined together in a latent church of the afflicted.

Guilt sends the alcoholic out into the original communities from which he fled, whose members he has aggrieved, offended, and injured, to repair wrongs. Shame forces him to join the altogether new community of similarly afflicted. There he needs to repair his own soul in a community which never excludes the self for reasons of its own shortfall. In AA, everyone has fallen short, has found himself lacking, has known despair and powerlessness, has seen the disapproving look in his child's eye or the even harsher disapproval in the eye of his own soul.

The Ecclesiology of the Movement. In addition to the Twelve Steps, AA and its spinoff organizations affirm Twelve Traditions.[32] The Twelve Traditions develop, in effect, the movement's "ecclesiology," its sense of appropriate organizational form. The Twelve Traditions resolutely reject the temptations to organize the community hierarchically and charismatically.

Traditions Two, Eight, and Nine specifically and unequivocally reject hierarchical authority: "Our leaders are but trusted servants, they do not govern." While "our service centers may employ special workers," the organization "should remain forever non-professional." Any service boards or committees created must be "directly responsible to those whom they serve."

AA also rejects the temptation to succumb to charismatic authority. An organization that relies heavily in its ritual of telling one's story might easily succumb to the spellbinder. But the very title of the organization warns against the charismatic: Alcoholics *Anonymous*. Tradition Twelve states: "Anonymity is the spiritual foundation of all our traditions, ever reminding us to place principles above personalities." Tradition Eleven specifically bans revealing identity to the media, the most likely vehicle for turning anonymous penitents into evangelizing personalities and celebrities. "We need always maintain personal anonymity at the level of press, radio, and films."

AA's opposition to both hierarchical and charismatic authority derives ultimately from the movement's knowledge of the alcoholic's deepest problem: his loss of self-esteem. The alcoholic suffers from feeling his own worthlessness and therefore tends to depend on and resent more powerful figures. To the degree that he pays attention to more powerful figures, the alcoholic loses a sense of his own direct access to transcendent power. His lack of self-esteem only increases. He feels cut off, unworthy, if others stand between him and lock him out by the assertion of hierarchical office or personal gifts. Only a nonhierarchical, noncharismatic community can let its members deal directly with their shame, restore their self-worth by experiencing sacred power directly.

When the powerless congregate—alcoholics with their fellow alcoholics—they offer each other a sense of direct access to transcendent power. In effect, the group permits each of its members to need and to lack, and thus clears the barricades that guilt and shame erect and creates an open space that allows an inrush of power. Thus the transcendent power of which the early movement speaks finds its home in the community of the needy. Despite their differences in language, both the religious and nonreligious alcoholic can work together; the religious speak of power, the secular of community. But both occupy the juncture where the vertical, power, and the horizontal, community, meet. As Bill Wilson put it, "our group strength seems to stem from our individual and ever potential weakness."[33]

Professional Expertise vs. Lay Experience. The American Medical Association initially reacted skeptically, and indeed contemptuously, to AA. In its review of *Alcoholics Anonymous,* the *Journal of the American Medical Association* (October 14, 1939) put down the Big Book as "a curious combination of organizing propaganda and religious exhortation. . . . The one valid thing in the book is the recognition of the seriousness of addiction to alcohol. Other than this, the Book has no scientific merit or interest."[34]

A more patronizing attitude eventually replaced this outright contempt. The medical community conceded that AA might sometimes succeed in treating or controlling symptoms, but asserted that the underlying problems that led to alcoholism needed the professional's intervention. (This concession ironically overlooked the fact that physicians could treat alcoholics only superficially and usually ineffectually. Pharmacological intervention, for example, could do little more than treat symptoms, and that at some price. The alcoholic might take Antabuse for help in keeping off the bottle, but, while on the drug, the patient suffered a convulsive, even dangerous, reaction to liquor.) Psychiatrists and analysts argued that only insight therapy could treat the disorder beneath the symptom, however effective AA might be in controlling the symptom. AA itself came to realize that members needed to do more than control symptoms. Bill Wilson identified "the dry alcoholic," the person who could abstain from drinking but who still thought like a drinking alcoholic. The dry drunk tends "to entertain grandiose plans and expectations, to nurse feelings of resentment, etc."[35]

A more sympathetic appreciation of AA appeared in the comments of Dr. Harry M. Tiebout, a psychiatrist, and Dr. E. M. Jellinek, founder of the Yale School of Alcoholic Studies (1943).[36] Dr. Tiebout notes that alcoholism may well be a symptom, but the symptom becomes a disease in its own right and, when rampant, blocks the therapist from dealing with other problems. Insomnia provides an analogy. Sleeplessness may result from a deeper disorder, but unless one can treat sleeplessness one may not be able to free the patient for deeper levels of intervention. This line of interpretation may simply value AA for providing important, albeit preliminary and superficial, help which prepares the patient for the long-term aid which the professional, working with the cooperative patient, can supply.

The distinction between these two levels of aid corresponds roughly to that already noted in the chapter on the battered between external behavior modification and fundamental long-term insight therapy. The former curbs destructive behavior; the latter tries to make deeper changes in identity.

Alcoholics Anonymous hardly breaks with medical practice. The movement interprets alcoholism as a disease. One of its founders was a physician; the other founder and one of its indefatigable apostles, Marty Mann, regularly sought treatment from Dr. Tiebout. However, AA does not define itself as subservient to the medical profession. While it sees itself as supplementing rather than contesting the medical establishment, it does not model itself on parent-teachers associations or hospital aides. It began treating not those cases the doctor was too busy to treat but those he could not handle—the hard cases that medicine could not touch. Members of the movement, even while calling alcoholism a disease, have often vividly and personally felt the limitations of medicine (and other professions) in curing it. The perceived inadequacy of doctors shows up dramatically in that AA ritual which most resembles the priest's confessional and the analyst's couch: the telling of one's story.

Why not tell one's story to a priest or a therapist who could offer comparable anonymity? Why tell it to a community of storytellers? "Elpenor" answers that question slyly: "We alcoholics are intensely social, constantly threatened by loneliness: we need to go out, mix it up with the crowd, see and be seen, perform. What can an audience of one do for us?"[37] While charming, Elpenor's explanation hardly accounts for the necessity of sharing one's story with this particular group. Performers need an audience, but an audience does not guarantee a performance that tells the truth. Indeed, for the sake of impact on their audiences, performers regularly trim and shave, expand and color their stories. The audience of fellow alcoholics must offer the storyteller something that he cannot find in a professional auditor. That something leads us back to the distinction with which this book began, the distinction between professional expertise and lay experience.

The expert relies chiefly on insight. Professional power differs from other kinds of power in that it derives from knowledge. This knowledge, largely universal, public, and abstract, applies handily to concrete cases. The expert may, as when prescribing drugs, apply this knowledge to the patient (who does not participate in the knowledge base), in which case the patient ignorantly benefits from it. Or the expert may, as in insight therapy, help the patient acquire abstract knowledge and, through that learning, change his behavior. In either case, the professional begins with and deals from abstract and general knowledge.

AA explicitly rejects this approach in favor of the alcoholic's immediate and individual experience. Insight will not do the job. "The actual or potential alcoholic will be unable to stop drinking on the basis of self-knowledge. This is a point that we wish to emphasize and reemphasize."[38] Help needs more power than knowledge offers. "The defense against the first drink must come from a higher power."[39] Convinced that alcoholism flags a deeper problem, the professional analyst seeks a cure in the form of an answer to the question, why? The analyst assumes that answering that question will lift a rock and let a cleansing light pour in and will dry out the patient.

AA cuts across the intricate analyses which psychotherapists offer with a terse warning: "Keep it simple." Like behavior modifiers, AA emphasizes beginning with externals, that is, with actions that precede understanding. "Just bring the body to a meeting and the mind will follow." Or again, "Act your way into good thinking. You don't think your way into good actions in this program."[40] Neither injunction suggests that thought doesn't matter. It just will not trigger the spring for saving action.

The action that precedes thought, which AA calls for, differs from the strategies of the experts, and does not distance the patient from lay experience. In fact, it bombards him with the importance of going to the meeting. There, he and his fellows will ponder the Twelve Steps and listen to one another's stories, sharing insight and thus treating their disease more deeply than could experts, by sharing a knowledge born of experience. This experience comes through ordeal. It emerges, as W. Jackson Bate put it, "ex periculo," out of peril. In the course of that peril, the alcoholic reckons with himself as weak and powerless but discovers, as he tells his story in the midst of the similarly afflicted, a strength born of weakness. Thus "a recovered alcoholic can reach and treat a fellow sufferer as no one else can." The expert who was himself a victim and thus could judge both abstract knowledge and particular experience concedes the superiority of experience over expertise. Dr. Bob reports on the first exchange with Bill: "Of far more importance was the fact that he was the first living human being with whom I had ever talked, who knew what he was talking about in regard to alcoholism from actual experience. In other words, he talked my language."[41]

Today the medical establishment and AA treat each other cordially.[42] The largest string of alcohol and substance abuse clinics in the country, run by the Lutheran General Health Care System, seeks to cooperate actively with Alcoholics Anonymous. An expert who works for the clinics contrasted the roles of the professional and the lay movement and revealed how much conventional expert attitudes have changed. Initially professionals tended to see the work of lay support groups as stopgap, temporary measures that waited upon professional treatment programs to produce more enduring change. But the professional now accepts AA's own reverse picture of the relative values of professional expertise and experiential healing. The professional at best can offer only temporary help, stopgap and transient. "My patients don't remember their counselor's name." But AA membership creates a fellowship that changes one's enduring identity. It defines a way of life.

Politics supplies us with an analogy for this last assessment. Monarchy treats citizenship as transient, in contrast to the perduring office of the king. "Long live the King!" The royal office, replete with power, endures. A Republic, the American Revolutionary thinkers argued, reverses the relative power, status, and endurance of the magistrate and the citizen. A Republic treats magistracy as the strictly temporary, and citizenship as the truly permanent and indelible office which all its members enjoy. Something akin to citizenship obtains in the polity of the self-help groups whose members benefit transiently from the ministrations of professionals but who even more enduringly require that identity which they receive and assimilate through the experience of mutual support. It is not accidental that AA began in the United States, a Republic, a citizen's democracy, at least in its ideal.

OTHER TYPES OF SUPPORT GROUPS

Three types of support groups have developed in response to the needs of patients and their families coping with illnesses resulting from addiction, from disease, or from stressful transitions in life. The support groups dealing with addiction, such as Narcotics Anonymous, Gamblers Anonymous, Sex Addicts Anonymous, and Overeaters Anonymous, tend to pattern after AA. The meetings are highly structured, tend to follow the pattern of the Twelve Steps, and deal with, among other problems, questions of the members' guilt and shame.

Support groups of the second type help members cope with diseases, such as Alzheimer's, cancer, or cardiovascular conditions leading to a stroke or a heart attack, or with such therapeutic rigors as a colostomy or renal dialysis. Members of groups of this type are less disposed to state their problems existentially or religiously. Guilt and shame will less likely figure as immediate issues. Members will orient more practically to the group for support, friendship, and information. In some cases, the group, such as the National Alliance for the Mentally Ill, will also engage in political action and public advocacy.

Support groups of the third type include persons facing a particular ordeal that has no medical name. Carol Madison, director of the Dallas Self-Help Clearinghouse, has broadly characterized such persons as "people in transition." Support groups have developed, for example, for Parents Without Partners, for Grandparents Raising Grandchildren, and for members of blended families, the Stepfamily Association of America, Inc. (In Boston, of all places, a support group has developed for Mistresses Anonymous.) Resembling groups of the second type, groups of this type engage varyingly in support, friendship, information, and, in some instances, political action. Both types conduct less structured meetings than AA. The AA, for example, somewhat stringently prohibits other members from making critical comments or suggestions following a member's statement. But mutual support groups of the second and third types will permit and even encourage such "cross talk" in the course of a meeting.

A compiler of *The Self-Help Sourcebook*, Edward J. Madara, has offered general advice on starting and sustaining a mutual support group. The *Sourcebook* supplies down-home advice on such matters as "Don't Re-invent the Wheel," "Think Mutual Help from the Start," "Find a Suitable Meeting Place and Time," "Publicizing and Running Your First Public Meeting," and "Future Meetings." Eventually, the group will need to attend to such matters as group purposes, a membership, meeting format, phone networking, use of professionals, group projects, and strategies for dealing with group "highs and lows." Since professionals have begun an estimated one-third of all mutual support groups, Madara offers "ten steps" for professionals, many of them designed to help professionals empower the group and restrain themselves from domineering as they learn to serve as consultants rather than leaders.

Similarities do appear across all three types of support groups. Organizationally, they recognize the power of the affliction to set apart members and their families from others in the community who do not share their common experience. Within the group, they eschew hierarchy. They prize equality. While appreciating professionals and whatever contributions they can make, they recognize the need for members and their families to support and sustain each other in the midst of extended ordeals. While members of types two and three may orient more practically, and less autobiographically, to one another than those who suffer from addiction, still, shared experience and the community it creates, not just problem-solving, give the groups a kind of therapeutic power among their members. As the saying puts it, "misery loves company and company lessens misery."

Similarities appear in the problems faced by members of the several types of groups even on those points where the types seem most opposed. The so-called self-induced problems of addiction do not appear to be wholly self-induced. A physical component of genetic disposition apparently figures in the problems of the alcoholic and the obese. Meanwhile, the most straightforward victims of catastrophe may suffer from problems of guilt and shame, the problems of those more obviously complicit in their own maladies. The accident victim may fear that he belongs to those tagged "accident prone." The embarrassed look on the face of someone who has taken a spill reminds us that an untoward event can trigger shame even when the victim has not contributed to his upending. Genetic anomalies can send mates scurrying back up the family tree to find out who is "at fault" for the misfortune. And sophistication about preventive medicine has lengthened the lists of diseases which we must now consider self-induced or at least partly self-induced.

Further, the humiliating physical impacts of some diseases and their treatments produce a sense of guilt or shame however little one may have contributed to the onset of the disease. The male on renal dialysis for kidney failure or on drugs for hypertension struggles with the problem of impotence. The stroke victim suffers from depression. The patient with a colostomy must deal with problems in hygiene that he thought solved at the age of three. Finally, the rehabilitation programs for many diseases make stringent demands upon energy and time and require changes in outlook and identity that place heroic burdens on the shoulders of the unheroic. The demands can provoke in patients a nagging sense of failure and shortfall, as they attempt to take hold of their reconstructed lives. Members of all three types of mutual support groups, wounded healers of every stripe, can share the tranquilizing message and advice of the AA: one day at a time.

I would not want to claim that AA has influenced in all particulars the various mutual support movements that have proliferated in the past fifty years, nor that it should serve as the standard by which we invariably measure them, nor that it has solved all its problems. Some chapters of AA (and the Rational Recovery group explicitly) altogether forgo the religious tonality imparted by AA's founders. Many mutual support groups offer temporary, purely instrumental help rather than an existential redefinition of the self. And recent research on alcoholism suggests that complete abstinence may not offer the only route to a re-constituted life. All mutual support movements, moreover, face the temptation that every missionary society sooner or later faces; that is, the temptation to convert others in order to stay converted oneself. In yielding to that temptation, the missionary instrumentalizes others to make good on his own agenda. And yet, in its own perverse way, this temptation proves that the helper assists not as a self-sufficient monad but as himself afflicted and needy, the converted needs the unconverted as much as the unconverted needs the conversion. This mutual needi-ness awkwardly proves that we find no psychiatrists, doctors, or law-yers, no self-sufficient monads, in either Eden or heaven.

THE AFFLICTED
ASSISTING
THE AFFLICTED
Organ Donations for Transplants

MUTUAL ASSISTANCE in which the afflicted assist the afflicted includes not only patient and family support groups, such as Alcoholics Anonymous and the American Association of Kidney Patients, but also that further assistance which modern technology places within reach—the donation of body parts. Recent technical advances that have made possible successful transplants include ventilators that keep the organs of brain-dead people in suitable condition for transplantation, techniques for preserving the organs in the interval between extraction and delivery, and the development of immunosuppressive drugs that let the needy new host accept the organ on friendly terms. These advances have created new treatments for heart, kidney, corneal, and liver diseases, and perhaps imminently for Parkinson's disease, diabetes, and many other afflictions.

But moral and religious problems emerged, along with the technological advances, which needed resolution to produce an adequate supply of organs and in ways befitting our traditions. The uncertain status of the brain-dead person on the ventilator posed the first problem: Is the person living or dead? If living, then, to remove his vital organs kills him. The philanthropic deed rests on an act of assisted suicide or murder. The second problem bore on the status of the newly dead body. Even if one can medically justify pronouncing the brain-dead person dead, do the attitudes of awe, respect, and dread before the newly dead place obstacles in the way of cutting up the dead, albeit for a noble

purpose? And if not obstacles, do these attitudes at least establish constraints upon the choice of the method by which a society secures organs for transplantation?

THE STATUS OF THE
BRAIN-DEAD PERSON

Traditionally, the doctor declared a person dead when he or she suffered
an irreversible cessation of circulatory and respiratory functions. Brain
death (that is, the irreversible cessation of all functions of the brain,
including the brainstem) would normally and rapidly result in the collapse of the respiratory and circulatory systems. But the ventilator can
respire for the brain-dead person and keep the heart and lungs pump-
ing. Do these ventilator-assisted "vital signs," this continuing life in
parts of the body, mean that the person is alive?

To this day, the Japanese have tended to answer yes. The Buddhist
philosopher Takeshi Umehara deems the extraction of organs from the
brain-dead person an act of murder.[1] The Japanese bioethicist Rihito
Kimura wryly observes that the import of donor organs constitutes one
of the few items in which Japan suffers a trade deficit.

The United States has reached the opposite conclusion. As early
as 1968, an ad hoc committee of the Harvard Medical School recommended adopting new criteria for determining death so as to cover cases
of brain death.[2] In 1972, the Task Force on Death and Dying at the Hastings Center[3] reviewed and recommended approval of the Harvard criteria on the grounds that the Harvard Report did not redefine death
but rather adjusted the criteria for determining death. Dr. Leon Kass
of the Hastings Task Force argued that, traditionally, no one has ever
defined death as the *death of the whole organism* (life still continues in
parts of the body), but rather as the *death of the organism as a whole*.
The organism as a whole dies when the whole brain, including the
brainstem, ceases to function. Under this condition, the persistence of
life in parts of the body—the heart, the lungs, the kidneys, and the
liver—with the mechanical assist of a ventilator does not mean that
the organism can function as a whole. The patient (however much technology may have obscured it) is dead, and dead in no other way than
the tradition has ordinarily defined it, not as the death of the organism
in all its parts, but as a whole. This essentially conservative position
led the Hastings Task Force to concur with the Harvard Report.

The Hastings Task Force, however, rejected one of the several reasons that the Harvard Committee gave for developing the new criteria,
namely, the need for organs. A declaration of death should rest wholly
on the patient's condition and not on the needs of others for organs,

however pressing those needs may be. One should judge the patient dead only because the patient is dead and not because other users of organs are hovering nearby.

To invoke the need for organs as a reason for declaring a specific class of people dead creates a runaway, imperial argument, difficult to limit. Under the press of one kind of exigency or another, one could redefine death to include anencephalics, and then perhaps, next time, hydrocephalics, microcephalics, and so on, denying any independent and firm boundaries to mark off the dead from the dying or the vegetating. (Just such a pressure developed in the late 1980s. Some interest developed in equating death with the absence or loss of higher brain function, a determination which would define anencephalics, and some others, as suitable sources of tissue for transplantation.)

An opportunistic redefinition of death would eventually produce other unfortunate results. It would lead patients to distrust doctors and hospitals, and would weaken the readiness of families to donate the organs of truly dead patients. Convenience and utility should not justify enlarging the kingdom of the dead. While, historically, the need for organs and the development of the technology for perfusing and successfully transplanting them supplied the *occasion* for reflection on the criteria for determining death, the need for healthy organs should not influence the standards for determining that a patient or a class of patients is dead. That decision should rest solely on the patient's condition.

Once having reached this conclusion, the Hastings Center Report argued that the way is clear, assuming donor consent, to extract organs for the purpose of transplantation. While the need for organs should not serve as a *reason* for elasticizing the criteria for determining brain death, once these criteria have been legally established and correctly applied in a particular case, one should not feel morally inhibited about seeking consent for organ donations. Since the Task Force on Death and Dying issued its report, all fifty states in the United States have adopted the criteria through the vehicle of a Uniform Determination of Death Act (UDDA) or variants thereof on the basis of which transplants can occur in the United States.[4]

THE STATUS OF THE NEWLY DEAD BODY

Maigret suddenly realized that there was one character in the drama about whom almost nothing was known, the dead man himself. From the outset, he had been to all of them merely a dismembered corpse. It was an odd fact that the Chief Superintendent had often noticed before, that people did not respond in the same way to parts of a body found scattered as to a whole corpse. They did not feel pity in the same degree, or even revulsion. It was as though the dead person were somehow dehumanized, almost an object of ridicule.[5]

The clear-cut and independent determination of death does not remove all obstacles to organ transplantation. The newly dead generate feelings of awe, respect, and dread in survivors, and families traditionally have responsibility for the fitting disposition of the remains. Funeral rites express that respect for the dead, and those rites largely derive from religious tradition. The rites vary: Jews and Christians usually bury; the Buddhists cremate. But they all recoil from harsh treatment of the corpse. Thus a system for securing tissue must contend with the powerful and complicated emotions that death and the newly dead generate. The quotation from Simenon's novel *Maigret and the Headless Corpse* highlights one such complication. Extracting organs from a corpse at least partly dismembers it, and, as Simenon observes, dismembering violates; it dehumanizes; it reduces the body to an object of ridicule.

While a person lives, we identify him so profoundly with his body as to render the dignity of the two inseparable. Apparently this identity of the self with its body does not terminate abruptly with death. Admittedly, the corpse is no longer the person. And yet—while the body retains its recognizable form—even in death, it commands respect. No longer a human presence, it yet reminds us of that presence which once permeated it.

This complex tie unravels, however, argues Simenon, when the body loses its integrity. The detached organ or member becomes vulnerable to ridicule. It has lost its *raison d'etre* and thus its centeredness. It has become an eccentricity, an embarrassment, an obscenity. Even while failing to remind us effectively of what has vanished, it commits the indecency of not itself vanishing. A further severance now crazily compounds the original severance of death and leaves the community charged with picking up leftovers rather than laying remains to rest.

Proposals, then, for dismembering bodies, even when they serve important social purposes such as organ transplantation, awaken deep resistance. This reservation grows out of an aversion to, a shuddering at, the harsh treatment of a corpse. This aversion does not abate just because the carving will serve another's life. Thus, tellingly, a British brochure, offering advice on approaches to the family of the newly deceased, suggests, "It is usually preferable that an approach for organ donation in general be made rather than requests for specific organs."[6] The brochure advisedly urges keeping the request vague to avoid reminding the family too sharply of the eventual dismembering. Other brochures reassure the reader that the procedure will not disfigure the body. The cutter will treat the body "with respect and reverence." Such reassurances show the powerful need to avoid offending sentiment and to adapt appeals for organs to our sense of a fitting discharge of our responsibilities to the dead.

FOUR SYSTEMS FOR
SECURING ORGANS

Organ Donation. The Anglo-American world relies on a program of individual giving. Organ donation depends upon securing the consent of the donor in advance of death or the donor's family at the time of death. The driver's license bureau and the emergency room of a hospital provide the likely sites and times for such commitments. Appeals in such settings do not usually address persons as members of particular religious traditions, but as members of the indeterminate public at large. Thus they understandably invoke the general moral principle of beneficence, in the hope that individuals will overcome their reticence or aversion and seek to do some good for others.

A system that relies on individual giving has the great advantage of respecting the basic authority and responsibility that individuals and their families bear for the disposition of the dead. The Anglo-American tradition has invested the family with quasi property rights in the body of the deceased as a way of locating and protecting that responsibility. A program of individual giving acknowledges that breaks in custom or practice should occur only as the donor and the donor's family "opt in" with their consent.

Individual giving, however, has not generated enough organs for transplantation. The waiting list for organs (kidneys, hearts, livers, hearts/lungs, pancreases, and lungs) has grown from 8,000 in 1987 to 18,000 in 1989. The United Network for Organ Sharing (UNOS)[7] receives 1,400 to 1,500 additions to the waiting list each month. Many factors may contribute to the shortfall. While the UDDA and the Uniform Anatomical Gift Act (UAGA) have made organ donations legally permissible, general appeals to the moral principle of doing good may lack the power to overcome procrastination, apathy, or aversion. The decision to donate requires thinking about death or coming to terms with the death of a family member. Death seems too remote as one receives or renews a driver's license and too immediate in the emergency room of a hospital. The occasion passes by, either too abstract or too discomfiting. In any event, the inadequate supply of organs has created fresh pressures for a review of the various other methods by which one might obtain (and distribute) tissue and a review of the moral and religious conditions that support or oppose these various systems.

Some moralists have urged that we supplement the first method of securing organs with a second, the marketplace option of buying and selling organs. Still other moralists urge that we routinely salvage organs and other tissue, based on a doctrine of so-called presumed consent (which would let the society take organs from the dead except for explicit refusals from potential donors or their families). A final option deserves attention: a program of organized giving through the good offices of churches and synagogues, whose traditions still provide the setting in which many people come to terms with death and whose officials still conduct most funeral services in the West.

Buying and Selling Organs. The second method of securing organs, through the marketplace transaction of buying and selling, has received increasing attention. At the 1989 International Conference on Organ Transplantation at Ottawa, Canada, some commentators asked: What is wrong with the sale of organs? The marketplace, after all, is an efficient mechanism for distributing a huge variety of goods and burdens. Why not rely on the marketplace to increase incentives and thereby enlarge the supply of usable human body parts? The option of buying and selling has the further advantage of still vesting the responsibility for decisions about the body in the individual and the family. It merely extends their power to include sale as well as gift. It would enlarge the family's property rights in the body from *quasi* to *full* and let it dispose of organs and tissue as it deemed fit.

The theoretical ground for my objection to buying and selling organs has already been covered in the discussion of the Baby M case. The marketplace offers an excellent mechanism for exchanging goods and services within its appropriate sphere, but we debase the meaning of some goods when we put them up for sale. When we bribe judges, buy babies, or purchase prizes intended to honor excellence, we corrupt the meaning of the good so purchased. For this reason, the law wisely restricts the family to quasi rather than full property rights in the body of the deceased. This prohibition affirms that the human race trespasses an important boundary when, either on the national or the international market, it cuts up the body for sale. Such a marketplace respects no boundaries. Neither the body as a whole nor any of its parts is tinged with the sacred. A thing has whatever worth someone is willing to pay for it. I concede that an individual might be willing to sell blood or an organ for moral and even noble reasons—for example, to generate money needed by others whom the seller chooses to help. But the nobility of a particular act of selling does not redeem the tawdriness of a social system that would reduce a straitened individual to that kind of action. A society that would exploit the penurious to sell a part of themselves demeans itself and its members and fails to solve its problems fittingly. The desperately ill ought not to solve their health care needs through the desperately poor.

At the Ottawa Conference, some speakers sought to soften the differences between a commercial sale and an outright gift by proposing a system that would allow for a "rewarded gift." As a participant at the Congress, I argued against the latter proposal by observing that if a donor receives a financial reward only if he gives the gift, the transaction differs very little from an outright sale. Whether rewarded gift or sale, the marketplace fails to respect the human meaning of the body and the awesomeness of its demise.

Routine Salvaging or Presumed Consent. Under a program of individual giving, the donor or the family must "opt in" with its consent. Under a program of routine salvaging, the donor or family must "opt out"; otherwise the government can presume consent. A system of presumed consent prevails in fourteen European countries, all of them under civil law, rather than common law, traditions. In general, members of the society in common law countries tend to retain all rights and powers not specifically granted to the state. In civil law countries, the state holds all powers except those it specifically grants to citizens. Some commentators have seen a "fit" between systems of "opting in," the requirement in common law countries, and systems of "opting out," the legal provision in civil law countries. However, at the level of practice, the two different types of societies do not differ as strikingly as the contrast would suggest. Physicians in countries that presume consent still approach deferentially members of the family before proceeding with the extraction of organs from a deceased relative. Thus a system of "opting in" generally prevails despite the formal differences in the law.

However, in view of the shortage of organs, why not brush aside requirements for consent (and the counsels of deference and tact in seeking that consent)? Why not automatically take organs from the newly dead as the most efficient way of supplying the needs of those dying for want of an organ? Let atavistic emotions about violating the body give way to reason's moral demand. What bearing does a rather primitive emotion, an instinctive aversion or revulsion, have on the resolution of a modern policy issue?

Recently, philosopher Joel Feinberg has joined those who back routine salvaging. While conceding that the bereaved might react emotionally to the routine cutting up of a corpse (which still symbolizes the dead person), Feinberg argues that one should not sentimentalize the newly dead body at the expense of real "people out there suffering and dying."[8] The woman who weeps over an episode of suffering on the stage but neglects it the next moment in real life symbolizes for Feinberg an objectionable preference for the aesthetic over the moral, the emotional over the rational. Since people are suffering and dying for the lack of organs, sentiment should yield to reason. Our aversion to cutting up a corpse should give way to a "careful rational superintendency, an education and discipline of the feelings."[9]

This chapter attempts to explore candidly some of the profound aversions people feel toward giving their organs or the organs of their kin for transplants. These aversions complexly trace back to our attitudes toward the newly dead and the funeral practices we have developed to express (but also contain and shape) those attitudes. Respect for these aversions, in my judgment, argues against a system of routine salvaging of organs.

Organized Giving. Yet, in arguing for the fourth option, a system of organized giving, I do not propose that our sentiments and symbols should escape criticism. Feelings are neither infallible nor inviolable, least of all those surrounding death. Our propensity to shudder at the thought of cutting up Uncle George, even for the sake of organ transplants, does not automatically rule out all other considerations. Indeed, no one could seriously propose the organized giving of organs and other tissue who did not believe that we should discipline and direct our feelings.

But reason does not provide us with the sole means for disciplining our feelings. Religious symbols (and the rites by which we appropriate them) can help express but also contain and discipline our most powerful feelings. Indeed, religious symbols and rites may strengthen, much more than appeals to reason, our capacity to secure organ donations, because religious communities, not simply reason, shape our attitudes toward death and most rites surrounding death. Thus this chapter must include a review of religious beliefs and practices that both oppose and provide positive reasons for organized giving. While religious communities offer a huge potential for organized giving, we must persuade them of its importance on religious grounds.

SENTIMENTS, RITES, AND SYMBOLS

Some students of funeral practices have pointed out that flight characterizes the most primitive human response to a corpse. Flight reflects more than an instinctive hygiene or an individual aversion to a dead body. Entire villages have been known to move to another location to avoid any further contact with a corpse. This powerful human aversion, however, did not escape discipline. Funeral practices arose, at least partly, as a way in which the community could contain and appropriate the horror. Analysts today have come to respect the psychological necessity of such rites. The living can pass on to mature life only through death and through consent to death. The Jungian Edgar Herzog concludes from dream analysis that the arrested adult fails to mature because he cannot participate in the final "killing" of his parents, an act which carries with it the responsibility to assume his parents' role. In taking their place, he must admit to being an adult who in his own time and place must die. In refusing to "kill," that is, to bury, he reveals that he fears dying and thus is unready to live. The arrested adult must pass through death to life.

The development of funeral rites therefore represents a secondary response of containment on the part of the community to force itself to be present to death. It does not allow raw feeling alone to drive it. The community must discipline its aversion. It must still its feet, as it were, and stay with the deceased. This form of presence, of course, does not wholly eliminate the original aversion. The community becomes present, after all, for the purpose of removal. It burns or buries the corpse. The community no longer journeys away from the dead, but sends the dead on a journey, as it were, away from the community. The original element of aversion and horror persists even within the containing form of funeral practice.

The modern humanitarian will grow impatient with this kind of analysis. What bearing does a rather primitive emotion like horror have on the humane resolution of a modern policy issue? Yet horror may have more bearing on our humanity than it appears. We may pursue unwisely the worthy policy goal of organ transplants by sidestepping or repressing the fact of aversion in the choice of means.

The Grimm Brothers story cited in the chapter on the molested warns against dismissing the importance of revulsion in personal life. It may also bear on developing responsive institutional practices. The young hero of the story is incapable of horror. He does not shrink from the dead—from either a hanged man he encounters or a corpse with which he attempts to play. From one point of view, his behavior seems pleasantly childish, but, from another, subhuman. Ashamed of him, his father sends the young man away "to learn how to shudder." Not until he has learned to shudder will he emerge from his nameless, undifferentiated state and become human. At a somewhat more comic level, the modern undertaker has difficulty securing respect for his person and work because of his over-familiarity with death. Our laughter and disdain testify to our deep sense of the connection between human dignity and a capacity for dread.

A policy that institutes the routine cutting up of corpses, even for high-minded social purposes, may fail precisely at this point: its refusal to acknowledge the fact of human horror. A tinge of the inhuman marks the humanitarianism of those who believe that social need easily overrides all other considerations and would reduce cutting up our dead to everyday, casual routine. Even the proponents of routine salvaging concede indirectly the awkward fact of human revulsion when they argue that routine salvaging spares a hospital staff the necessity of making "ghoulish" overtures to the dying patient or to his relatives. Perhaps, however, a society that overrides rather than faces up to profound reservations imposes on them, more ghoulishly.

Human horror before death does not remain a formless, unspecified emotion. The object of horror links with images and symbols that in turn associate with institutions. Specifically, we have noted that death links in the imagination with the acts of hiding and devouring. The routine salvaging of organs particularly tends to fix on the hospital an association with death as devourer. A breakdown in health has already produced in the patient a sense that the world has exhausted and consumed all his resources. The hospital traditionally offered a respite from a devouring world and the possiblity of recuperation. However, the high cost of modern health care and aggressive treatments increasingly associate the hospital itself with devouring. A system of routine salvaging of organs would merely confirm that process of devouring. Upon the patient's death, the state would now cut out, package, and distribute his organs on behalf of the society. What is left over is utterly unusable husk.

While the procedure of routine salvaging may, in the short run, furnish more organs for transplants, in the long run it would depress and corrode that trust upon which the arts of healing depend.

A system of salvaging that requires the donor's consent and/or the family's consent respects, for want of a better phrase, what Jacques Maritain once called the principle of the extraterritoriality of the person. The person's final transcendence of the state undergirds the family's traditional legal rights concerning burial. This respect for transcendence does not confine itself to common law countries. Sophocles' *Antigone* expressed eloquently the conviction that no other party could normally interpose claims upon the corpse that would interfere with the family's right and obligation to provide for a fitting disposition of the remains. In other words, whatever use and abuse, conflicts and tragedies, a person has suffered in the course of his public life, the society cannot reduce him to those ragged events alone. Antigone insists that she has a duty and therefore a right to bury her brother Polyneices, despite the king's wishes in the matter. In defying the king and insisting on a proper burial, Antigone claims that her brother transcends the social order. In covering him over with the "thirsty dust," she signifies that the state cannot fully devour him.

Does extraterritoriality adhere to the person, or to his family? Must an Antigone bury a Polyneices because he is a *man*, or because he is her *brother*? The first question asks the meaning of a funeral service for any and all families. In pursuing the latter question, we will have to cope with further ramifications for the subject of organ transplants.

From one perspective, the burial service presupposes and reinforces the continuity between the person, his mortal remains, and the family unit. This continuity remains particularly strong while the newly dead body maintains its recognizable form; it weakens when the body returns to particles. So viewed, funeral rites express the continuity of the soul with its body and with the gathered community of friends, colleagues, and family. From this perspective, the principle of extraterritoriality applies to the family group. The corpse, the deceased, and the family belong, as it were, to a continuum which should enjoy sanctuary against the larger society and the state. Given this sensibility, if one wanted to proceed beyond traditional funeral rites to a justification for donating organs, then one would need to interpret the donation as a further and different expression of continuity between the generations. Something like Robert Jay Lifton's—or preceding him, Unamuno's, Soloviev's, or Bulgakov's—concept of symbolic or surrogate immortality would then shape the funeral service and the donation of organs.

From a different perspective, the funeral service, far from maintaining continuity with the deceased, publicly acknowledges that death has shattered that continuity. Intimates whose lives have inextricably intertwined now need to acknowledge a break. The family especially needs these rites of surrender. "Dust thou art and unto dust thou dost return." Nothing so forces the community to acknowledge that the process of separation has begun as the rigidity of death and the finality of cremation or burial. From this second perspective, one will view the decision to proceed beyond traditional funeral practice and donate organs to the living not as a way of achieving symbolic immortality but as a finite act in which one mortal human being assists another.

This second perspective also argues intensively against a system of routine salvaging of organs, because routine salvaging places the burden of initiative on the family to seek exemption from the state's right of eminent domain. Placing this burden on the family wrongly and indecorously forces the family to *claim the body as its possession*, but only in order to proceed with rites in the course of which it must acknowledge surrender and separation. Antigone has a right to bitterness in her contest with Creon. She must claim her brother's body as *her* possession—not Creon's—precisely at the moment when death forces all concerned to recognize a human being beyond their grasp.

Society has wisely vested "quasi property rights," directed to a decent burial, in the family, because the family, most of all, must acknowledge that he has moved beyond its effective control. The rites tacitly acknowledge that the deceased is now what he has always been, a human presence whose extraterritoriality must be honored.

Thus, the provision of organs for transplants should preferably rest on a system of consent. If one grants the state the comprehensive authority to dispose of the corpse, or package it as it pleases, then a society has traveled a long way toward conceding to the state total and unlimited control over the person, living or dead. Funeral rites, which center on the "remains" attended to by the family and intimates, help establish the principle of a reality above and beyond the claims of the family and the state. Precisely those who have most cultivated and consumed the person in the course of his living—his family, colleagues, and friends —those who have most eaten him alive, and whom, therefore, loss, guilt, and remorse most afflict need to acknowledge his final transcendence. If he provides yet another meal for others in death, that act of love should be freely elected.

Now we must return to Joel Feinberg's criticism. Have we respected the fact of human aversion toward death but fallen into the opposite trap of sentimentalizing sentiment and rendering untouchable the corpse and unchangeable the rites and procedures from deathbed to burial and cremation? I think not. For funeral rites, as we have seen, do not themselves leave raw emotion untouched. Funeral rites themselves have already contained and disciplined the original, raw impulse to avoid and flee. This containment of original feeling comes at a great price, however, and generates its own heightened level of sentiment, specifically an aversion to any and all who would interfere with the rights and duties that go with that tie. This sentiment lies behind the protestations of Antigone and the wariness of Gypsies who hover around a hospital deathbed to make sure that nothing untoward happens to the corpse; and it generates the quasi property rights to the body in Anglo-American law.

I would hardly conclude, however, that sentiment should be left at its new level, wholly exempt from yet further discipline. Clearly, the very effort to mount arguments for organized giving of organs implies yet a further effort to shape and conform feeling. But the power of feeling argues that bland appeals to reason and to the general ideals of beneficence, altruism, and philanthropy will not suffice. We may need to appeal not simply to the superintendency of reason but to the religious traditions themselves and their shaping convictions and symbols to develop sufficiently powerful reasons, religious and moral, for securing organ donations.

Optimistic people once argued that an adequate supply of organs depended merely upon passing a Uniform Anatomical Gifts Act. But not all obstacles are *legal*. Indeterminate appeals to the public at large through media appeals and advertisements on buses and subways will not likely generate many donors. Purely individual appeals lack organizational momentum. They also address the *isolated* individual, one-on-one, exactly in that condition and circumstance which most resembles death itself—the individual, solitary and removed from community. To secure substantial support for organ and tissue donations one will have to go beyond a tepid legal permit and general appeals to individuals.

We must mobilize institutions, chiefly religious institutions, since they at least partly shape convictions about death and since most funerals still occur under religious auspices. Religious tradition offers an important resource for arousing conscience and for developing an institutionally directed program of organized giving.

RELIGIOUS ATTITUDES AND ORGANIZED GIVING

A survey of official religious groups on the subject of organ donations does not look too promising. A 1980 report[10] on sixty-nine denominations and traditions revealed, for the most part, either neutrality, mild approval, or inattention to the issue. I will not try to survey these various official denominations, but will explore, instead, five root religious attitudes and their implications for recovering human body parts.

At the far extremes, two religious outlooks oppose not only the specific techniques of organ transplantation but also the medical enterprise altogether. The first outlook, associated with the Christian Science tradition, is monistic, idealistic, and optimistic in tenor. The Christian Scientist holds to the reality of the spiritual realm and the ultimate unreality of the body, sickness, and death. Thus the Christian Science healer must help the patient achieve a transcendent spiritual perspective that will dissolve the apparent power of disease, rather than distract the patient with medical interventions or reconstructions of matter that lack ultimate significance.

At the other extreme lurks a religious dualism. This dualism does not shape an official, extant, religious tradition today but it marks our culture in its more pessimistic strains. Such dualism traces back to the ancient Manichaeans who divided all reality into two rival powers: the Kingdom of God, associated with Absolute Spirit and the Good; and the Kingdom of Satan, associated with Absolute Evil and Matter. The world we live in hopelessly confuses Good and Evil, Spirit and Matter; salvation depends upon escape from this messy and disspiriting confusion. Thus the early Manichaeans opposed sex, marriage, and procreation (sex is bad but kids are worse), and, to be consistent about it, any therapeutic measures designed to prolong our stay in this essentially evil world. The symbol system is strange, but it persists in modern behavior. The ancient Manichaean and the modern pessimist find little warrant for bringing children into the world or for prolonging, through medicine, one's stay in a world that has lost its savor. In his last public interview as he reached his eighties, the former head of the draft, General Hershey, said, "I don't see too good and I don't hear too good, but there isn't much to see or hear."

A third type of religious outlook—a variant of optimism—traces back to the ancient Gnostics (the Greek word for knowledge). The dualistic mythology of the Gnostics distinguished sharply between spirit and body. The mythology has long since faded; but its outlook persists in the modern world in the dualist philosophy of René Descartes. The Gnostics effectively anticipated one of the most powerful attitudes in modern culture—the assumption that salvation will come through knowledge. This confidence in saving knowledge provides, in its secular form today, handsome support for the modern research university, its professional schools, and the technologies that university research has helped produce. We look chiefly today to the professional's knowledge-based power to provide the means for altering and improving the given world. For Gnostics, ancient and modern, the body is not so much unreal or evil, but incidental. Technology treats nature as incidental raw material to be converted into miracle drugs and wonder products.

The Gnostics were also religious dualists; but they believed that the spirit and the body are loosely, rather than tragically, tied to one another. One seeks through knowledge to surpass the ordinary limitations of life in the body. This general outlook, linked with the good intentions of modern technology, provides a spiritual basis for the strategy of routine salvaging of organs and other materials from the body. Since the human identity with the body is incidental, one need not seek permission from the predeceased or from the family for extracting, in a good cause, organs, blood, or tissue. There is no rational reason why salvaging should not become routine, except for the provision of procedures to exempt the recalcitrant. (I would associate the obtaining of organs through buying and selling with no religious view but rather with a wholly secularized and secularizing marketplace which reduces all things to assets for sale.)

A fourth religious attitude—a variant of pessimism—does not view the world and the human body as evil, but perceives human life to be in the grips of evil and destructive powers. Evil forces rather than good powers rule the universe; they are random, multiple, and destructive rather than creative and nurturant. Modern medicine operates largely within this generally demonic understanding of disease. Sickness results not from the withdrawal of a positive, lifegiving power (the ancient shaman's *animus*) but from the invasion of negative and predatory forces (the germ theory of disease). We live in an age beset by evils; we largely think of ourselves as hostage to impersonal forces that will eventually do us in.

Within the confines of this religious vision we can adopt only two strategies: resistance and avoidance. We can resist those powers that threaten to destroy us (hence the drive behind the health care system in our time to fight unconditionally against death); or we can seek to avoid death (hence the temptation of staff and friends to withhold the full truth from the stricken and the dying). These two responses of resistance and avoidance create the crisis we face in organ donations. The strategy of resistance heightens the demand for ever more organs for transplants to stave off death. But reflexive avoidance makes it extremely difficult to get individuals to donate their organs to further that fight. Signing that donor card requires them to reckon with the fact that they will one day die. Thus avoidance dodges what resistance demands.

The fifth religious attitude—the Judeo-Christian tradition—has officially dominated the West. As opposed to the Christian Scientists and other idealists, this tradition views the body as real rather than unreal; as opposed to the Manichaeans, it affirms the body as good rather than evil, worthy of preserving. Both affirmations converge to justify medical treatments, including transplants. But, as opposed to the Gnostics, the tradition affirms a profound link and identity of the spirit with its somatic existence; thus it would not be as ready as the Gnostic to justify invasions of the body, living or dead, without explicit consent and it would reject a strategy that would reduce the body to an asset for sale. The religious tradition would generally opt for a system based on giving rather than routine salvaging or selling.

Beyond this point of agreement, the Jewish and Christian traditions deserve individual treatment on the subject of organ transplants. While Jewish law generally prohibits mutilating a corpse or delaying its burial, an urgent need to save a particular life suffices to override this prohibition. Judaism, generally, recognizes the right to use body parts to save lives, assuming, of course, that the donor's death has been clearly established.

In the following, however, I will concentrate on Christianity, both for reasons of competence but also because the Christian Church remains a major institution in the West, with significance for millions. Not that the Christian tradition could or should be legislatively decisive on the subject. The Christian tradition no longer occupies an official, regulative position in Western life and culture. Law based on Christian ethics alone would be divisive (and therefore objectionable even on Christian grounds). On the other hand, its attitude on the subject could have considerable impact on the success of a system of blood donation and organ and tissue retrieval. Thus we need to examine closely potential obstacles and warrants for procuring organs in the light of Christian thought and practice.

An important feature of traditional Christian teaching—the doctrine of the resurrection of the body—seems to forbid or discourage organ transplants. Christian expectations for future life were not dreamy and spiritual. Christians looked forward to a future life as bodily life together in the presence of God. Given these views of future life, early Christians favored the custom of burial, rather than the total obliteration of the corpse through cremation.

Does or should Christian belief in bodily resurrection throw barriers in the way of a new kind of destruction of the body—not through cremation but through the extraction of organs from the corpse? I think not. As Augustine observed, burial is not a *condition* of the resurrection, as though God were somehow prevented from accomplishing his purposes with those who were smashed to pieces or incinerated. Burial, he asserts, is "no aid to salvation," but "an office of humanity,"[11] Burial simply testifies fittingly to the resurrection; it declares that the faith does not condemn the body or devalue it to the status of a disposable cartridge.

This argument, however, does not carry us very far. It merely removes an obstacle; it does not, of itself, provide positive reasons for the extraction of organs from the corpse. Does the Church merely acquiesce to such procedures reluctantly, that is, merely permit them, or does the faith provide its own positive moral and liturgical reasons for this act of giving?

Morally, the Christian looks to Christ for his or her understanding of God and the moral imperatives which that understanding entails. Self-expending love defines Jesus' life—he lays down his life for the brother and the sister, the neighbor, the enemy and the stranger. This self-donative love both defines the Son of God and impels the Christian to love the neighbor. Scripture makes it clear that this love calls for concrete service to the bodily needs of others—their hunger, thirst, and illness. (To prevent sacrifice from masking masochistic behavior, this service to others has its customary Christian limits in two provisos: the sacrifice must have some chance of success in helping others, and the sacrificer must ordinarily not neglect those duties to himself or herself that will sustain a future capacity to serve.)

Christian liturgy, as well, provides a powerful, specific reason for donating one's own body. Christians believe that, in the sacrament of the Lord's Supper, Christ shares, under the form of bread and wine, his body and blood with his disciples. He invites and bids his followers to share in his self-giving love. Fittingly and directly, believers may participate in this worship by their readiness to share a portion of their bodies and blood with others.

While Christian ethics and worship justify and encourage organ transplants, the Christian, I suspect, would have to draw back from the sentimental and inflationary language of some who would want to interpret such deeds as acts ensuring symbolic immortality. "My child died in the accident, yet he lives on by supplying others with a heart and a kidney." Such deeds themselves, for the Christian, cannot confer immortality or divinity; they signify God's self-donative love, which they themselves cannot reproduce. The language of symbolic immortality exaggerates too much for Christian monotheists. They should rather talk simply about the assistance that one mortal being renders another.

Further, the receiving of an organ does not rescue the living from the need to die. The gift only defers the day when the recipient will have to do his own dying. Nor does receiving an organ, in and of itself, teach the living how to live—unless the recipient, in receiving the organ, discerns a self-donative love of which the giving of the organ may be a modest sign. No sentimental excesses, please, in the direction of symbolic immortality.

If Christian ethics authorizes the giving of one's organs, nerve, bone, blood, and skin to unknown recipients, does it eliminate the need in such cases to hold funeral services? Has the liturgy already taken place in the hospital? What about the gutted remains? I would suggest on this point that Christians might consider an analogy again from their chief sacrament.

In current eucharistic practice the Catholic and Episcopal churches and others have developed customs for the respectful disposition of the leftover consecrated elements. The priest either keeps them in the tabernacle—the so-called reserved sacrament—takes the remaining elements to the sick, consumes them, or pours them into the ground. It is inappropriate to flush them down the toilet. This respect toward leftover bread and wine has some bearing on the ceremonial disposition of those bodies from which we have extracted organs. Rites should provide for the respectful disposition of the remains of remains which have served as the matter of a fraternal action within the human community. Such ritual provision is hardly a condition of salvation, but it testifies to the privileged place of the body in acts of love.

Christians who take seriously these moral and liturgical warrants for organ transplants will need to organize and collaborate with others to these ends. Individual appeals made to individuals at the driver's license bureau or late appeals to families in the emergency rooms of hospitals will secure some organs, but hardly enough. Ministers and priests will need to prepare their congregations long in advance of crisis and help them perceive that the donated heart beats not only with life but with love.

Despite these reasons for Christian giving, religious communities have still not organized as fully as they might.

ANENCEPHALICS, ABORTED FETUSES, AND THE JUST DISTRIBUTION OF TRANSPLANTS

Meanwhile, further issues have emerged in securing organs and fairly distributing them. Should we take organs and other tissue, upon parental consent, from anencephalic babies or from aborted fetuses? How should we distribute gifts? To fellow citizens only? To only those who can privately pay for the additional medical costs of transplantation and implantation? Will failing to satisfy the canons of justice in the distribution of gifts weaken programs of organized giving?

Anencephalic Transplants. According to estimates, we need in the USA 400–500 infant hearts and kidneys and 500–1,000 livers a year to meet the needs of children currently dying of these diseased organs. Since children (as opposed to teenagers) do not die accidentally in sufficient numbers to meet this need, some experts have looked to anencephalics as a potential source of lifesaving organs.

Even if we could resolve all the theoretical moral issues, Dr. D. Alan Shewman of the UCLA Medical Center has questioned whether using anencephalics as sources of transplant organs would materially help to meet the need.[12] In the USA an average of 1,125 anencephalics are born every year. Nine hundred survive screening and elective abortion. Among these, the 600 stillborn shrink the pool to 304 live births of which 122 are large enough to supply organs. Probably only two-thirds (80) of the parents of these anencephalics will consent to donate. Current success rates in transplants would probably yield no kidneys, 9 hearts, and 2 livers. In ten years, assuming improvements, particularly in kidney transplants, Dr. Shewman expects 25 kidneys, 12 hearts, and 7 livers that would benefit their recipients. Dr. Shewman urges that we bear in mind this small yield "before we expend great effort in modifying diagnostic criteria for brain death, changing statutory definitions of death, or relaxing fundamental principles of transplantation ethics in order to obtain anencephalic organs."[13]

The theoretical question still remains. Would a greater yield of transplants justify changes in the diagnostic criteria for determining brain death or in the principles governing transplantation ethics? For the reasons developed in the earlier discussion of brain death, I would oppose redefining death for reasons of need. The state of New Jersey has considered (New Jersey Assembly Bill No. 33677) the alternative route to securing organs from anencephalics by amending, not the UDDA, but the Uniform Anatomical Gift Act (UAGA) to permit taking organs from a special class of patients (anencephalics) not yet dead. This proposal evinces the virtue of honesty since it does not blur the distinction between the living and the dead. But Professor Alexander Capron and other critics have opposed it. Capron argues that we should not choose the most vulnerable of living donors for sacrifice. However imperfect anencephalics may be, they do result from the "live birth of the product of a human conception";[14] we cannot claim that they are not human. The tragedy of an anencephalic pregnancy also opens the door to manipulating the parents. Thus recruiters might suggest to parents that they will partially redeem the pregnancy by not aborting or by choosing a caesarean section for the sake of producing mature and healthy organs.

Capron also surmises that the long-term cause of organ donations would suffer from this aggressive proposal. The worry that this amendment to the UAGA might lead to yet further encroachments upon other vulnerable groups might, in fact, surround the UAGA with general distrust and generate additional legal resistance that would cut down the supply of organs from heretofore eligible groups. He concludes, "Medical ingenuity should be directed toward finding ways to care for dying anencephalic (and other) babies so that when they become brain dead they can be organ donors with their parent's permission."[15] Until that time, moralist Gilbert Meilaender urges, "Our obligation is not to achieve all the good we can, as if our responsibilities were godlike. It is, rather, to effect all the good that we can within the limits morality places upon us. Not only what we accomplish but what we do counts."[16]

Fetal transplants. The potential pressure of need and demand on the 1.5 million abortions per year in the USA vastly exceeds the pressure upon and possible use of anencephalics. Over one-half million people suffer from Parkinson's disease (60,000 new cases a year in the USA) and one-half million people from diabetes who might benefit, if research succeeds (some view that success as problematic in the case of Parkinson's disease), from fetal transplants of brain tissue and pancreatic tissue respectively. John A. Robertson has pointed out that "Nearly 80 percent of induced abortions are performed between the sixth and eleventh weeks of gestation, at which time neural and other tissue is sufficiently developed to be retrieved and transplanted. Abortions performed at fourteen to sixteen weeks provide pancreatic tissue used in pancreatic transplants, but it may eventually prove possible to use pancreases retrieved earlier."[17] Others foresee uses of fetal transplants in the treatment of other disorders. The list of possible treatable diseases and injuries includes Huntington's chorea, Alzheimer's disease, spinal cord injury, cortical blindness, bone marrow failure, sickle cell anemia, leukemia, aplastic leukemia, thalassemia, and hemophilia. Robert Stevenson, president of the Tissue Culture Association, has testified that the potential medical value of tissue culture from fetuses far surpasses the medical value of whole, adult organs secured from conventional donors.[18] The long, fibrous axons in older brain tissue makes fetal brain tissue the most suitable for transplantation. The often pathologically compromised tissue of fetuses from spontaneous abortions makes tissue from elective abortions the most suitable source.

The general prohibitions in the UAGA forbid securing organs from live, nonviable fetuses or paying for the tissue itself (as distinct from paying the medical costs of extracting, transporting, and transplanting tissue). For the reasons adduced earlier in this essay, I would oppose paying for fetal tissue, whether directly or indirectly (through the payment for the abortions). The latter policy issue may not remain hypothetical if the Supreme Court decision of July 3, 1989 in the *Reproductive Health Services v. Webster* case leads to more restrictive laws making it more difficult for poor women to secure abortions. The federal government already prohibits the funding of abortions, and more and more hospitals depend upon federal funding. Further, laws of the kind that the state of Illinois is considering at this writing, which would require clinics performing abortions to maintain expensive, hospital-level equipment, will dramatically increase the cost of abortions and place them beyond the reach of the poor. Were some states to adopt further restrictions against abortions in private facilities, women would need to travel to other states to secure an abortion. Women, poor or modestly fixed, may be increasingly tempted to sell the fetal tissue to pay for the abortion. This possibility does not argue for lifting the prohibition against the sale of fetal tissue but for considering carefully the recent directions in our basic policies on abortion.

Several issues remain. Should one restrict the source of tissue to spontaneous (as distinct from elective) abortions? If one uses elective abortions, should the law restrict the pool to fetuses from ectopic pregnancies or, more broadly, to fetuses independently elected for abortion but not extend to fetuses expressly aborted for purposes of transplantation?

The fetus in an ectopic pregnancy is likely to be normal, more mature, and wanted by the parents, but unable to survive without killing the mother. Donations approved by parents in this case avoid the special moral difficulties of using the unwanted aborted fetus and would conform to normal patterns of giving upon death of a child.

The law, in my judgment, should prohibit taking and using fetal tissue from a woman who became pregnant for that express purpose or who, once pregnant, aborted an otherwise wanted child to provide fetal tissue. Both practices, though surely rare, would convert the acts of conceiving, gestating, and delivering a child into manufacturing and ought to be prohibited. Since, however, the law cannot deal satisfactorily with motives, this prohibition can take practical form only by prohibiting the donation (or sale) of fetal tissue to an identifiable party. Such a prohibition would spare a woman the pressures that might bear down on her when faced with the needs of a particular person.

What then of other abortions in which the child is unwanted? Absolute pro-choicers would not object to securing from the mother consent to use tissue from her fetus. Other, less absolute, pro-choicers, recognizing the tragic element in the decision, would balk at using fetal material from an elective abortion as a first resort. Kathleen Nolan expressed this view when she said, "Being used once is enough."[19]

Pro-lifers also divide into two camps. The majority undoubtedly would prohibit both elective abortion and any following effort to secure and use the fetal tissue. Fr. James Burtchaell has argued that the woman who has elected to abort forfeits the normal rights and duties of parental guardianship and therefore the right to make a gift of the remains. The fetus has died, not by accident, but by parental choice. Using such fetal tissue, absolute pro-lifers believe, resembles using knowledge gained from experiments in Nazi concentration camps. It establishes retroactively a kind of complicity, a "supportive alliance," to use Fr. Burtchaell's phrase, in evil.[20]

Critics of this majority view argue that using fetal tissue available through the evil of an abortion is not, of itself, evil, unless one has urged or supported the original abortion. John Robertson, himself no pro-lifer, illustrates this principle (to which a small minority of pro-lifers might subscribe) by pointing out that using the organs taken from a murder victim does not of itself make the transplant surgeon or the beneficiary an accomplice to the original killing or encourage subsequent acts of murder.

The supporting analogies for this criticism—Nazi atrocities and homicide—do not strike me as entirely apt. First, the original deeds do not compare in moral gravity. The painful, sometimes tragic decision to abort does not compare with either Nazi atrocities or the act of homicide. Pro-choicers would emphasize this dissimilarity. Many pro-lifers, however, would emphasize a second dissimilarity. They see a much stronger connection or "supportive alliance" between the subsequent use of fetal tissue and an originally elected abortion than obtains between beneficiaries and original agents in the analogies. The current use of knowledge gained from Nazi atrocities, some fifty years in the past, does not derive benefit from an extant system; the use of fetal tissue does. One cannot, in the latter instance, so tidily separate the two sets of agents. No single agent spans the original event of homicide and the subsequent use of tissue from a homicide victim. (The only bridge figure, the deceased, is supremely patient rather than agent in both cases.) In abortion/donation, however, the parent acts as agent both in aborting and in deciding to give the fetal tissue. Perhaps this complication led Kathleen Nolan not to oppose the use of electively aborted fetal tissue but to use it (a) only as a last resort (after exhausting the supply of fetal tissue from ectopic pregnancies) and (b) with the understanding that the term "gift" does not describe the moral status of the tissue supplied. One has simply "contributed" what, for one reason or another, one already does not want.

While always ready to concede the importance of language, I am not sure that the lowering of moral resonance from "gift" to "contribution" makes that much difference in the resolution of this issue. Moreover, "unwanted" does not begin to describe the pregnant woman's complex feelings toward the fetus. While choosing abortion, she is not usually insensitive to the pain of that decision.

The Human Fetal Tissue Transplantation Research Panel of the National Institutes of Health (December 1988) either heard as testimony, or itself generated, most of these arguments. Its report concluded, but not unanimously, that fetal tissue, with appropriate safeguards, should be made available for research. Those safeguards should insulate as much as possible the decision to abort from the decision to use the fetal tissue. Neither the researcher nor the recipient should play a role in counseling to abort or in performing the abortion. The woman should not be approached for her consent to contribute tissue until after she has made the decision to abort, to avoid manipulating either that decision or the timing of its execution (to produce, for example, a more mature fetus). Current prohibitions against selling the abortus or designating a particular party as its recipient should also remain in force. Even with these safeguards in place, three members of the panel opposed the final recommendations. At this writing, the Bush administration has refused to act favorably on the majority's recommendation.

Clearly, willingness to approve or to oppose the use in transplantation of fetal tissue from elective abortions has turned largely, though not absolutely, on the attitude toward abortion itself. Although the NIH panel sought not to repeat the debate over abortion in reaching its recommendations, judgments on that issue affected conclusions.

The U.S. Supreme Court, at the time of this writing, seems to be referring the question of abortion policy back to the several state legislatures. Pro-choicers fear what the states may do to prohibit abortions altogether. Some states, however, might possibly opt for a more unconditional pro-choice position that would eliminate the *Roe v. Wade* trimester distinctions between early and late abortions. The Court's distinctions, acknowledging the legal importance of the different stages of fetal development, rest on a morally important point. The *Roe v. Wade* decision implied that we obscure the moral issue by using the univocal term "abortion," with its associated moral evaluation, to cover the entire nine months of fetal development. Early and late abortions resemble one another less than early abortion resembles contraception and the abortion of a developed fetus, infanticide.

Thus we may need to take care not to lump together and univocally approve or disapprove the use of human tissue from all electively aborted fetuses, whatever their stage of development. A more developmental view, of course, makes it difficult to draw lines. But neurologists such as Dr. Julius Korein have remarked that, at 19–20 weeks, synapses develop in the cortex. Once synapses develop, cerebral reticular formation takes place rapidly, wake/sleep cycles begin, and the organism soon can live outside the womb. To prohibit using fetal tissue from an elective abortion at or beyond 19–20 weeks may seem like drawing a fine line, not yet needed with *Roe v. Wade* still in place. But on just such fine lines civilized life depends. After 20 weeks, we abort, not just a potential, but an actual, human being.

Distributing Organs Justly. The problem of commercializing transplants does not hinge solely on whether we secure organs by purchase or gift. The organ itself may be a gift, but the system by which we extract, preserve, transport, and implant organs may be so expensive and market-driven as to pose serious questions of justice, not in their acquisition, but in their distribution. Dr. Carl Kjellstrand of Stockholm and the University of Minnesota[21] has offered evidence that in the lineup to receive organs for transplantation, men go before women, the young before the old, whites before blacks, and the rich before the poor, and in percentages for which medical/biological factors cannot account.

We do not distribute organs fairly. An unjust system of distributing organs, in addition to being intrinsically wrong, also compromises efforts to secure organs. One can hardly, for example, solicit gifts of organs from all, including the poor, if the delivery system discriminatingly deposits them in the bodies of the rich. In Washington, D.C., for example, "during 1982–83, approximately one-fourth of the 125 transplanted cadaver kidneys went to non-immigrant aliens, often Saudis whose religion prohibited mutilation of the corpse for organ removal."[22] One would not want to support a chauvinistic policy that refused organs to foreigners, but one may reasonably infer that such outcomes in Washington, D.C. resulted not simply from a generosity toward the non-immigrant alien but also from a marketplace deference to the rich.

Decisions in the so-called "micro" allocation of scarce lifesaving resources should conform to the general guidelines which James Childress[23] proposed long ago for allocating the then scarce resource of kidney machines: physicians should first determine medically those who most need and might benefit from treatment; and, when the number of medically qualified patients exceeds available resources (in 1981, for example, the 2,150 usable cadaver kidneys fell far short of the need of 7,000 to 10,000 dialysis patients waiting for renal transplants), our health care system should randomly distribute the treatment, without regard to the race, color, creed, national origin, or social contributions of the recipient. Professor Childress has more recently adjusted these policy proposals to deal with the special circumstance of patients in need of organ transplants.[24] A system that depends upon love in the production of a good ought not to fall below the level of justice in its distribution.

The recently established United Network for Organ Sharing has attempted to solve the problem of treating foreign nationals justly by allowing them to register, like any American, for a national waiting list. This procedure would eliminate earlier local abuses, such as letting them jump the queue by paying more money. Further, U.S. government funds could not be used to pay for their transplants. While recognizing that some cities, by virtue of demographics, handle a larger number of foreign nationals petitioning for transplants (for example, Washington, D.C.), UNOS monitors those cities and institutions where the number exceeds 10 percent of the total.

Ultimately, however, the "micro" question concerning the fair distribution of particular organs does not compare with the "macro" question of how much money the society should invest in such expensive, acute care treatments. Should we, for example, spend more money on liver transplants instead of increasing our allocations to prevent alcohol abuse? The USA has chronically and disproportionately spent money on acute care, instead of preventive medicine. Physicians brush aside such "macro" issues by arguing that further investments in acute care need not weaken support for preventive medicine. They suggest that we take the money, instead, from other parts of the federal budget, such as stealth bombers and the space program. This ploy, however, overlooks the other important social programs already queuing up for any freed-up funds. The USA already spends almost 12 percent of its GNP on health care, a commitment which far surpasses that of every other nation. The case is weak for reserving a still higher percentage of funds for acute care treatments.

Our ability, however, to live within current limits on funding may depend upon our capacity to limit the fear of death that currently distorts the budgetary priorities of Americans. Our fear of death has already bloated our commitment of public funds to the Defense Department and to the Department of Health and Human Services and, in the private sector, to health care fringe benefits for workers. This fear of death has generated the strategy of all-out resistance to death, and the pressure to secure organs by any means to keep alive any and all patients with life-threatening diseases.

The Western religious tradition, to the contrary, holds that human disease and suffering are real but not ultimate. The reality of the diseased kidney and the suffering it imposes justify the donation of organs and the medical interventions to implant them. Such resistance to death is natural. But, at the same time, human disease, suffering, and death are not ultimate. We should not sustain transplant policies driven by fear alone, supporting acute care medicine without limit, at the expense of preventive medicine and other human goods. We resist too desperately when we assume that the powers ruling the universe threaten and destroy, pure and simple. We lose that deeper ease about the human condition which would allow us to relieve distress but with a final metaphysical nonchalance. Only from that nonchalance can we relieve distress vigorously while accepting, without complacency, the moral limits upon our struggle against death. To reiterate Professor Meilaender's point: our own responsibilities are not "godlike," "our obligation is not to achieve all the good that we can . . ." but "to effect all the good that we can within the limits morality places upon us."[25]

POSTSCRIPT

AT THE CLOSE of the chapter on the Dax case, I suggested that the health care team cannot adopt the role of parent toward the patient, because members of the health care team have not, like parents, endured in their own time what they now ask the patient to endure. The victim of catastrophe has suffered an ordeal which the experts have not themselves directly experienced. The patient resembles not the child curled in the bosom of the family, but the hero in Greek tragedy whose affliction has cast him out beyond the safeties of hearth and city gates.

Clearly, Greek tragedy does not offer the only account of a human life pitched out beyond the pale. The Christian tradition finds its savior there. I have referred to that tradition only in passing; yet some reference appeared in each of the chapters. The Christian theme of death and rebirth inevitably shaped the discussion of the severely burned patient. That patient faced a terrifying baptism by fire in the catastrophe and a subsequent baptism by water in the Hubbard tank. The parents of the retarded undergo a similar ordeal of death and rebirth. Additionally, I noted in the discussions of the retarded and the gestated and sold that the dual responsibilities of parents for the being and well-being of their children reflect the Christian tradition on the two aspects of divine love: God's accepting love and his empowering love. The partly Christian notions of guilt and shame figured large in the discussions of battering and incest; further, the decision as to whether to help the batterer and the molester, as well as their victims, required some thought about the scope of the Christian responsibility for care. The chapter on the elderly dealt with the role of religious ritual in the formation of the virtues important in old age. My essay on total institutions demanded some attention to the religious context which must shape social action if it would not gratuitously afflict the afflicted. And the discussions of mutual support groups and organ donations dealt with Christian motives and forms for organized giving.

But I have not explicitly reckoned with the Christological reasons for these passing references. Inevitably, I need to close this book with a word about Jesus' solidarity with those whose stricken identity has been the subject of this book.

That solidarity dominates both the Scripture narratives and the creeds of the church. Unlike the ancient myths of the dying and rising savior whose bloody wounds magically flower into blossoms, the New Testament never softens aesthetically the reality of his ordeal. Jesus suffers prosaically. The nails are real. His risen body still bears the marks of his crucifixion. The earliest and the shortest of the Christian narratives, the gospel of Mark, spends fully one-third of its pages on the passion of Jesus. Mark and other of the gospel writers seize upon the suffering servant passages from the scriptures of Israel to interpret Jesus' ordeal. The passages from Isaiah place God's servant among the stricken. "As many were astonished at him . . . his appearance was so marred, beyond human semblance, and his form beyond that of the sons of men . . ." (Isaiah 52:14). Or again, ". . . he had no form or comeliness that we should look at him, and no beauty that we should desire him" (Isaiah 53:2b). The accounts in Isaiah place God's servant among the spiritually as well as the physically mangled. "He was despised and rejected by men; a man of sorrows, and acquainted with grief, and as one from whom men hide their faces he was despised, and we esteemed him not" (Isaiah 53:3).

The major creeds of the Christian Church unmistakably connect Jesus with the experience of tribulation delineated in the patient's ordeal and identify him, in turn, with God. The narrative accounts of the Incarnation which the creeds affirm trace the downward path of love from God to humankind in which God establishes total solidarity with men and women in their plight. The Apostle's Creed emphasizes not only Jesus' death and rebirth, but the specific details of the ordeal of death and rebirth that have shaped this essay. Jesus suffers death in all its dimensions: he undergoes the agony of separation from his flesh, community, and God. As the Creed puts it: he "suffered under Pontius Pilate, was crucified, dead, and buried; he descended into hell." Scripture fills in the details.

His death, like all others, separated him from his flesh. The narratives specify this ordeal factually, including the detail of dehydration. He suffered, first, dispossession and loss of control of his world: the king with no subjects, the teacher with no pupils, the healer who bleeds. He also endured severance from the world as savored. His world effectively dwindles in his last hours to a sop of vinegar, the darkened sky, and a spear in the side. He also suffered, like all other men and women before and after him, the final stiffening of the expressive body in the unrevealing mask of the corpse.

His death also separated him from community. One sees this separation at work beforehand in the persecution by the high priest, the ambiguities of the Roman governor, the fickleness of the crowds, the betrayal by Judas, the cowardice of Peter, and the sleepiness of laggard followers in Gethsemane. This separation from community culminates in the final, definitive exclusion of his burial.

Jesus suffers finally the ultimate tribulation, which men and women have never fully faced, the absence of God. Inasmuch as men and women have never fully honored the presence of God, they have not fully suffered the terror of God's absence. They nestle in some corner of the creation and let it cradle them, order them, soothe them, and stimulate them, until catastrophe strikes and dislodges them from their snug little home in the world, for which disconcerting ordeal we reserve the term *anomie*. But these traumas of separation serve only as prologue and sign of the ultimate, dimly perceived terror of God's absence. As the Creed puts it, he descended into hell.

Men and women fear separation from their flesh because they manage and savor life in and through their flesh. They fear separation from community because they become human only in and through their community. They fear the disruption of the tempo and rhythms of their familiar world, because, absent those rhythms, all else goes awry. But what are these fears compared with the most terrifying of them all, separation from God, who grounds life in the flesh, the community, and the world? This question remains partly rhetorical for other men and women inasmuch as they know only partly what they ask. But God's absence and separation reinforce all other separations for Jesus, who, as the Son of God, descends into the region that stands under the blank terror of the absence of God and yet holds fast before God, through God, and for all people. Suffering God's absence, he yet prays to the Father, the absent God present through the lips and ordeal of his Son. "Father into thy hands, I commit my spirit" (Luke 23:46).

The Christian tradition affirms that Jesus' solidarity with God and humankind frees men and women from ultimate tribulation. They need no longer stare in the mirror, worrying about the inevitable defeat of their flesh, or plunge into communities, worried about exclusion at their hands, or lift up their eyes to heaven, attempting in a blind fury of good works to force the presence of God rather than participating freely in his power and attending to his will. For the Savior who identifies, soul and body, with men and women in his descent remains their Lord in his ascent to sustain them—bodily, together, in the presence of God.

So goes the Creed. But this affirmation hardly frees those who take it seriously from tribulation. After all, the prospect of rebirth conflicts in countless ways with all the terms and conditions under which men and women like to handle their lives. Entering into this new life also effectively confronts them as death, a death to their former selves. They can never reduce this new life to something added to their old aspirations and ideals. It perforce shocks them and rocks them. It surely imposes upon them an ordeal, which the older theological tradition sought to acknowledge under the notion of purgatory—that temporal interim in the midst of eternity wherein the not yet fully salvaged soul must still reckon with eternal life as a death. But death, in this second meaning of the term, does not annihilate; "it destroys [but] only in the interest of bringing forth in us a new identity."[1]

Ordinarily, this new identity does not take hold in the instant. As the chapters on the burned, the retarded, the battered, and the molested make clear, a complex, continuing struggle between identities ensues. The "old man" and the new life contest daily and diversely for the soul. Luther expressed and compressed the complexity of this struggle in the religious life when he referred to the Christian as "saved, sinner, and repentant" at one and the same time. If Luther's formulation described only a temporal progression, he would have had to refer to the three in the obviously chronological order: sinner, repentant, and saved. Luther recognized, however, that the person of faith does not live the new life by simple possession, the old life utterly dead; he thus resorted to the language of simultaneity—saved, sinner, and repentant.

This untidy state of affairs might suggest that nothing has really happened, that the stricken self continues to thrash and flounder. The change, however, is complex but real. Admittedly, one does not live the new life by simple possession; nevertheless, one lives it by direction and hope. Just so, the person on the way to healing does not wholly escape vulnerability and discouragement. But healing has mercifully begun to take hold.

Further, the emergent new identity is not itself devoid of death. Scripture insists that the risen body of Christ still bears the marks of his crucifixion. Self-expanding love—laying down one's life for others —is the abiding mark of this new identity. Thus men and women discover in Jesus' suffering and dying an identity which receives itself unceasingly from God and spends itself unceasingly for others. Of this death, Arthur C. McGill writes: ". . . there there is nothing evil at all; on the contrary, this death is a *meal*. This death is a *festivity*."[2] In receiving this meal and acting on it, men and women participate in a love which freely lays down life for them and calls them similarly to expend themselves for their fellows.

This receiving and giving which the sacrament represents should radiate outward into the specific lives men and women lead and the sufferings they endure, as they imperfectly nourish and are nourished by one another. The afflicted assisting the afflicted, I have called it in this book. Eventually, the Christian burial service for each should testify to the ways in which he or she has participated in the dynamics of this giving/receiving love. The obituaries should, "in reviewing the life of every person . . . acknowledge how neediness has been filled by others. At the same time, an obituary [should] also record this person's life, that is, the course of his or her self-expenditure in the context of his or her dying."[3] This record of assisting and being assisted in the midst of need testifies to the way our wayward lives connect with the ultimate. It integrates death "within the rhythm of giving and receiving" which defines the triune life of God: the Father, Giver; the Son, Receiver; in the bond of the Spirit.[4]

Participating in this ultimate power that reveals itself in Jesus' suffering and death provides warrant for facing into all that men and women find negative, ugly, and ludicrous in human affairs without fearing their power to engulf. It should help create persons and institutions with the courage not to flee from their own neediness and therefore with the courage "to join the needy, to comfort them in affliction, to call them out of their despair, to countermand their fear."[5] But participation in this powerful love also posts its exclusions. Specifically, it undercuts the two great responses to suffering and death which tempt both modern medical practice and the modern church: a desperate avoidance and an equally desperate resistance to death. A final comment on the force of these exclusions brings this postscript and this book to a close.

The reflexes of avoidance and resistance have largely defined our perceptions of the physician's role as parent and fighter. The impulse to protect the patient from the crushing burden of disease and death has led to the definition of the physician as the overprotective parent who manages the truth and makes decisions on behalf of the patient.[6] Total institutions have also served paternalistically to buffer the society at large against a too-close contact with suffering and death. But the churches have similarly encouraged patterns of avoidance. Many persons report that they have never heard their minister or priest take up directly in a sermon any of the ordeals described in this book, never mind the question of their own dying. Thus preachers repeat and confirm those patterns of avoidance which the health care system offers. Still other clergy preach the resurrection in such a way as to attempt a verbal bypass around the reality of death. Thus the church blurts out, like the rest of the culture, that it has nothing to say about death, except "to say it with flowers."

To whatever degree the church avoids death, it betrays unconditionally the Christian message. It offers only a momentary respite from secret apprehensions, before death tricks or snatches each from the sanctuary into the graveyard. The church must preach about death if it would preach joyfully. Otherwise it speaks with the profound melancholy of men and women who have separated the church from the graveyard. It concedes the existence of two Lords. First, the Lord of the Sabbath, the God who presides over the affairs of cheerful Philistines while they still thrive and enjoy good health. Then, a second Lord, a Dark Power about which one never speaks, the Lord of highway wrecks, bedside squabbles, hospitals, jail houses, and graveyards who handles everything in the end.

The Christian faith, however, does not proclaim two parallel Lords. The Lord of the church does not rule a surface kingdom. His dominion is nothing if it does not go at least six feet deep. This conviction forms those terse statements about Jesus' career in the Apostle's Creed, "suffered under Pontius Pilate, was crucified, dead, and buried." The Creed thereby blocked the nonsense of those early theologians who wanted to deny the humanity of the savior or who speculated that he was merely asleep or resting between Good Friday and the resurrection morning. The church countered and insisted that he truly suffered and died. The testimony of scripture left the faith no other conclusion. God himself under the form of the Son had gone down into the grave.

This perception of God's solidarity with the suffering and dying also forbids a human response to disease and death defined wholly by a desperate resistance. An anxious resistance to death largely drives the broader civilizing activities of humankind, whether in the reproduction of the species, the military defense of nations, the pursuit of careers, the aspiration to command and power, the publication of books, the creation of fortunes, the creation of works of art, the naming of buildings, or the daily jostling for prestige. Men and women engage in these death-defying activities to silhouette themselves against a dark background. Anxious resistance to death is the dark underside of the human quest for immortality.[7]

This resistance also shows up intensively in those desperate efforts to combat disease and death which the modern physician organizes, playing now the role not of parent, but of fighter. This resistance sees no limit to the war against death and thus brooks no limit on treatment. It produces overtreatment and iatrogenic illness. It tempts people to continue fighting even when futile treatment only imposes more suffering on the host to the disease. It has pushed health care costs in the United States beyond 11 percent of the gross national product and it tempts the society to bury its defeats by sequestering the profoundly impaired-but-still-living in total institutions. This strategy of resistance often joins forces with the response of avoidance, as professional institutions, in collusion with the family, pretend that they can do more technically, refusing to concede that their ingenuity has reached its limit.

A society fears to respect that limit because it dreads religiously the nullity that yawns on the other side of it. But if the anointed of God, as Isaiah avers, has exposed himself to deprivation and oblivion and death, and yet flourishes and persists even there (and especially there), unceasingly receiving himself from God and unceasingly spending himself for others, then men and women need no longer fear that the negative which they see in others and perceive in themselves can separate them from God. God under the form of the servant has exhibited the powerfulness which is his, and ultimately ours, as receiving and giving love.

This ultimate religious optimism should not undercut the motive for works of mercy and relief and forthright efforts to resist evil and reform defective institutions. Religious hope should not lead to quietism and complacency. Rigorous social action need not depend upon a grim pessimism that sees life as a desperate struggle between humankind and the negative that assaults from without and corrodes from within. On the contrary, the recognition of God's ultimacy deprives the negative of its ultimacy and therefore frees physicians, nurses, patients, and families to do more confidently and faithfully what they can and spares them the responsibility and temptation of trying to do more than they can. Freed of the burden of messianism, they can perform whatever works of relief and tenderness they can and accept such works themselves from others, as a carefree sign of a huge love between them which they themselves have not produced.

However, this ultimate religious optimism, this final nonchalance, hardly persists in either care-givers or care-receivers without contest or trial. The Christian tradition recognized this struggle when it dealt with suffering as a test of faith. The abyss, the *anomie*, the impoverishment, and the pain that disease or accident imposes or the suffering of the innocent that retardation, battering, and molestation expose surely test one's convictions about the powers that rule human life. The word "test" only palely describes the tribulation which the person of faith suffers. What powers truly govern human life? Powers that ravage the mind, paralyze the will, benumb the sensibility, and corrupt the body? Or, powers that nurture, uphold, bless, and heal? In the midst of actual suffering, one can hardly answer that question *pro forma*, casually, or by simple repetition of slogans. As Job discovered, a change of identity must occur. Faith will either crack or it will deepen and grow; but, in either case, it is no longer the same. To appeal to the ordeal which the Dax case presents and with which scripture is acquainted (I Peter 1:6–7), fire changes the metal it tempers.

NOTES

Introduction

1. See Paul Ramsey, *The Patient as Person* (New Haven: Yale University Press, 1970), p. 122 for comments on the traditional Roman Catholic distinction between ordinary and extraordinary means.

2. Moralists, on the whole, would reject the suggestion that they have neglected the patient's plight. After all, ethicists have relentlessly criticized professionals across the past twenty years for their failure to respect the patient's autonomy. In arguing for that respect, moralists think of themselves as champions of the patient's moral dignity. However, ethicists do not adequately respect or protect the moral being of patients if they simply clear out a zone of indeterminate liberty free from medical interference but fail to lead the patient to discuss the moral uses to which the patient puts his liberty. They let the patient dwindle, in effect, to a bundle of wants and interests which can dispose of itself as it wills without answering to the wisdom of that disposition. Presumably, it suffices that the patient has made *his own* decision. *What* he decides or what behavior he displays is of little moral interest. Tipping one's hat to autonomy alone consigns the patient to moral oblivion. A liberty merely patronized is a moral being denied. Respect for the patient demands more than giving him leeway, licensing him to do, say, or be whatever he pleases. Respect must include a willingness to engage the patient and the patient's family in a moral give and take, a sometimes painful mutual deliberation, judgment, and criticism, and an occasional accounting for one another's views, on both sides, in the professional exchange.

3. For the value of Eliot's distinction in explaining the question of professional virtue, see William F. May, "The Virtues in a Professional Setting," Third Annual Memorial Lecture, The Society for Values in Higher Education, *Soundings: An Interdisciplinary Journal*, 1985.

4. W. Jackson Bate, *Samuel Johnson* (New York: Harcourt Brace Jovanovich, 1975), p. 297.

1. The Burned

1. See "DAX Case Revisited," an audiovisual tape, produced by Don Pasquella of Southern Methodist University, Dallas, TX, for all quotations from the Dax case. This tape used some material from the earlier clinical tape on the Dax case, not intended for general viewing: "Please Let Me Die," Videotape Library of Psychiatric Disorders, Vol. 129, May 1974.

2. Leslie E. Einfeldt, R.N., M.S., "A Preventive Nursing Approach from Injury to Recovery," in *Comprehensive Approaches to the Burned Person*, Norman R. Bernstein, M.D., and Martin C. Robson, M.D., eds. (New Hyde Park, NY: Medical Examination Publishing Co., Inc., 1983), p. 118.

3. See Martin C. Robson, M.D., "Reconstruction and Rehabilitation for

Admission: A Surgeon's Role at Each Phase," in *Comprehensive Approaches*, Bernstein and Robson, eds., for an account of the medical fight to deal with consequences of the skin's destruction.

4. Robson, "Reconstruction and Rehabilitation . . . ," p. 42.

5. David Bakan, *Disease, Pain, and Sacrifice* (Boston: Beacon Press, 1971), p. 32. The word inserted in the brackets is mine.

6. John D. Constable, M.D., "The Limitations of Aesthetic Reconstruction," in *Comprehensive Approaches*, Bernstein and Robson, eds., p. 285.

7. Ibid., p. 288.

8. Ibid., p. 285.

9. Nancy Hanson, R.P.T., "Practice and Planning in Physical Therapy," in *Comprehensive Approaches*, Bernstein and Robson, eds., p. 193.

10. "DAX Case Revisited," op. cit.

11. Arnold van Gennep, *Rites of Passage* (Chicago: The University of Chicago Press, 1972), and G. van der Leeuw, *Religion in Essence and Manifestation*, Vol. I, Ch. 22, "Sacred Life" (New York: Harper Torch Book, 1963).

12. Van der Leeuw, *Religion in Essence and Manifestation*, Vol. I, pp. 192–193.

13. William Shakespeare, *Henry IV*, Part II, Act V, Scene V, 52–53, 60–64. The Folger Library General Reader's Shakespeare, Pocket Books edition, 1961.

14. Wayne A. Meeks, *The Moral World of the First Christians* (Philadelphia: Westminster Press, 1986), p. 13.

15. See William Winslade, "Taken to the Limits: Pain, Identity and Self-transformation," in *Dax's Case: Essays in Medical Ethics and Human Meaning*, Lonnie Kliever, ed. (Dallas: Southern Methodist University Press, 1989), pp. 115–130, for an essay that emphasizes the continuities in Dax's self-transformation.

16. Fyodor Dostoievsky provides a literary example of the complexity of radical reconstruction and renewal in *Crime and Punishment*. The arrogant student and protagonist of the novel, Raskolnikov, aspires to the exercise of godlike power and kills for an abstract cause. At the end of the novel he repents, relents, and abases himself. At one level, no change in identity could be more radical than Raskolnikov's move from pride to compassion. And yet the shift in his character does not totally displace the old self. A foreshadowing of the new self appears earlier in Raskolnikov's repressed consciousness, in his dream life, and in some spontaneous acts of compassion. Only, however, after his conversion, his turning around, will the heretofore banished and marginal begin to order his life.

17. For details on Jesus' solidarity with the human loss of identity with body, community, and God, see the "Postscript" to this volume.

18. See William F. May, *The Physician's Covenant* (Philadelphia: Westminster Press, 1984), chapter 1, "The Parent," pp. 53–62.

19. This quote roughly paraphrases one of the surgeons in the Dax case, "DAX Case Revisited," op. cit.

20. Brian Clark's play *Whose Life Is It Anyway?* (New York: Dodd Mead, 1979) originally appeared as an audiovisual on the death and dying circuit, then evolved into a long-running London and New York play, and, at length, into a film. It dealt chiefly with the legal, not the moral, question as to whether the quadriplegic patient had a right to refuse treatment. For my views on that play and for an explanation of the distinctions between ordinary and extraordinary means, starting and stopping machines, allowing to die and killing for

mercy, see my chapter on the physician as "Fighter" (chapter 2) in *The Physician's Covenant*.

21. A. Napier Baker, "Pastoral Care," in *Comprehensive Approaches*, Bernstein and Robson, eds., p. 118.

2. *The Retarded*

1. For this and the following material on bonding, see Marshall A. Klaus and John H. Kennell, *Maternal-Infant Bonding* (St. Louis: C. V. Mosley, 1976), Chs. 1 and 3.

2. Ibid., p. 59.

3. Dr. Jerome Kagan has reported clinical evidence of these fears appearing at this age.

4. A. N. Solnit and M. H. Stark, "Mourning and the Birth of a Defective Child," *Psychoanalytic Study of the Child*, 16:523–537, 1961.

5. Klaus and Kennell, *Maternal-Infant Bonding*, p. 84.

6. Helen Featherstone, *A Difference in the Family* (New York: Basic Books, 1980), p. 25.

7. John Greenberg, *A Child Called Noah* (New York: Holt, Rinehart and Winston, 1972), p. 180.

8. For further details, see John Bowlby, *Attachment and Loss*, Vol. I (New York: Basic Books, 1969), p. 340.

9. See van Gennep, *Rites of Passage*, and Van der Leeuw, *Religion in Essence and Manifestation*, Vol. I, Part 2, Ch. 22, "Sacred Life."

10. J. Canning and C. Canning, *The Gift of Martha*, Children's Hospital Medical Center, cited by Helen Featherstone, *A Difference in the Family*, p. 220.

11. R. Massie and S. Massie, *Journey* (New York: Alfred A. Knopf, 1975), cited in Helen Featherstone, *A Difference in the Family*, p. 220.

12. Featherstone, *A Difference in the Family*, p. 220.

13. W. H. Auden offered this comment in personal conversation. I do not know whether he ever set it in print. This chapter on the retarded deals with the pressures that an immigrant nation's orientation to the achievement of its youth creates for the young; the chapter on the aged explores the corresponding neglect it encourages toward the elderly.

14. Featherstone, *A Difference in the Family*, p. 91.

15. Ibid., p. 188.

16. Sigmund Freud, *A General Introduction to Psychoanalysis* (New York: Permabooks, 1953). Freud writes: "What have we to do in order to bring what is unconscious in the patient into consciousness? At one time we thought that would be very simple; all we need do would be to identify this unconscious matter and then tell the patient what it was. However, we know already that that was a shortsighted mistake. Our knowledge of what is unconscious in him is not equivalent to his knowledge of it; when we tell him what we know he does not assimilate it *in place of* his own unconscious thoughts, but *alongside* of them, and very little has been changed." Twenty-seventh lecture, "Transference," pp. 443–444.

17. Klaus and Kennel, *Maternal-Infant Bonding*, pp. 86–94.

18. Featherstone, *A Difference in the Family*, p. 218.

19. Ibid., p. 166.

20. Leo Kramer, *A History of the Care and Study of the Mentally Retarded* (Springfield, IL: Charles C. Thomas, 1964), p. 7.

21. Featherstone, *A Difference in the Family*, pp. 213–214.

22. Ibid., p. 237.

23. Ibid., p. 220.

24. Ibid., p. 176.

25. Ibid., p. 10.

26. For the author's attempt to deal with the issue of theodicy, see the concluding comment to the chapter on "Afflicting the Afflicted: Total Institutions" and the "Postcript" to this book, in addition to the chapter on the "Covenanter" in May, *The Physician's Covenant*, Ch. 4.

27. Featherstone, *A Difference in the Family*, p. 83.

28. See the "Postscript" for a further discussion of the reciprocities of giving and receiving that define covenanted lives.

29. Søren Kierkegaard, *Fear and Trembling*, tr. Walter Lowrie (New York: Doubleday & Co., 1954), pp. 146–147.

30. Heidegger elevated the phrase *Sein zum Tode* (being-toward-death) into one of the fundamental categories of existence in his *Sein und Zeit* (Tübingen: Max Niemeyer Verlag, 1957), eighth printing, pp. 235–267.

31. Martin Buber writes, "God is the Being that is directly, most nearly, and lastingly, over against us." *I and Thou* (New York: Charles Scribner's Sons, 1958), pp. 80–81.

3. The Retarded Institutionalized

1. See the chapter on "Afflicting the Afflicted: Total Institutions" for further comments on deinstitutionalizing.

4. The Gestated and Sold

1. Thomas William Mayo, in "Medical Decision Making During a Surrogate Pregnancy," *Houston Law Review*, Vol. 25, Number 3, May 1988, provides a roundup of the 34 reports on the Baby M case in *The New York Times* alone.

2. See *In Re* Baby "M," 217 N.J. Super. 313, 525, A.2d 1128, 1142–43 (N.J. Super. Ct. Ch. Div. 1987) Aff'd in part and rev'd in part, No. A–39–87 (N.J. to Feb. 3, 1988).

3. George J. Annas, "Baby M: Babies (and Justice) for Sale," *Hastings Center Report*, June 1987, p. 15.

4. See Michael Walzer, *Spheres of Justice* (New York: Basic Books, 1983), pp. 97, 100–103, 282–283, for a discussion of the moral importance of blocked exchanges in curbing the tyranny of money.

5. Annas, "Baby M. . . ," p. 14.

6. Excerpts from the New Jersey Supreme Court decision "in the Matter of Baby M," *The New York Times*, February 4, 1988.

7. Apparently in the nine months following the Baby M trial court decision, some 70 bills bearing on surrogacy appeared before 27 state legislatures. See Peterson, "States Assess Surrogate Motherhood," *The New York Times*, Dec. 13, 1987, and Lori B. Andrews, "The Aftermath of Baby M: Proposed State Laws on Surrogate Motherhood," *Hastings Center Report*, Oct./Nov. 1987, pp. 31 and 38, as cited by Mayo, "Medical Decision Making. . . ," p. 603.

8. Samuel Johnson wrote the lines for Goldsmith's *Travellor*, cited by W. Jackson Bate, *Samuel Johnson* (New York: Harcourt Brace Jovanovich, 1975), p. 198.

9. Francis Kane, *The Evening Sun*, Baltimore, Thursday, October 5, 1989.

5. The Battered

1. The long account of the graduation ceremony does not appear in quotation marks because I took notes immediately following, rather than taped, the

meeting. However, the paraphrase follows as closely as possible the language, rhythm, and tone of the original meeting.

2. Texas Department of Human Services 1986 Annual Report, "Family Violence," p. 22.

3. Ibid., p. 21.

4. Ibid.

5. Ibid.

6. *Time*, "Private Violence," September 5, 1983, pp. 18–19.

7. Texas Department of Human Services, pp. 21–22.

8. See Texas Department of Human Resources Booklet, "Kids Should Be Seen and Not Hurt," August 1984. Stock Code 20561–0000.

9. W. H. Auden, "The Sea and the Mirror," in *The Collected Poetry of W. H. Auden* (New York: Random House, 1945), p. 357.

10. Roland A. Delattre writes, "The logic and dynamic of addiction is an ever-increasing dependence on an ever-narrowing source of reliable satisfaction —the increasing dependence showing from the need to escalate the dosage in order to receive the same level of satisfaction, together with an increasing incapacity to deal with other needs and alternative sources of satisfaction." Delattre, "The Culture of Procurement: Reflections on Addiction and the Dynamics of American Culture," in *Community in America: The Challenge of Habits of the Heart*, Charles H. Reynolds and Ralph V. Norman, eds. (Berkeley: University of California Press, 1988), Ch. 3.

11. One counselor recalls "a severely obsessive man—a high functioning CPA—who rigidly controlled all areas of his professional and personal life except for moments of psychotic-like rage when his wife pressed him for emotional intimacy."

12. Later research suggests that this particular rhythm of violence characterizes one type of violent man, not all. See Lenore Walker, *The Battered Woman* (New York: Harper and Row, 1977), p. 179.

13. Douglas K. Snyder and Lisa A. Fruchtman, "Differential Patterns of Wife Abuse: A Data-Based Typology," *Journal of Counseling and Clinical Psychology*, Vol. 49, No. 6 (1981), 878–885.

14. Ibid., p. 882.

15. Ibid., p. 884.

16. See Edward W. Gondolf, "Who Are Those Guys? Toward a Behavioral Typology of Batterers," in *Violence and Victims*, Vol. 3, No. 3, 1988 (Springer Publishing Company), pp. 187–203, and Daniel G. Saunders, "A Typology of Men Who Batter Their Wives: Three Types Derived from Cluster Analysis," unpublished paper, correspondence directed to Daniel Saunders, Family Service, 214 N. Hamilton St., Madison, WI 53703.

17. Sherry G. Lundberg, "Domestic Violence: A Psychodynamic Approach and Implications for Treatment," unpublished paper, Family Place Health Center—The HELP Center, Dallas, 13777 North Central Expressway, Suite 525, Dallas, TX 75243, pp. 10–11.

18. Ibid., p. 11.

19. See Maggie Scarf, *Unfinished Business* (Garden City, NY: Doubleday, 1980), for a popular account of the notion of unfinished business in diagnosis and therapy.

20. Daniel J. Sonkin, Ph.D., and Michael Durphy, M.D., *Learning to Live Without Violence: A Handbook for Men* (San Francisco: Volcano Press, 1982), appendix III.

21. Ibid.

22. Ibid., Ch. 5.

23. Dr. Herbert Benson, *The Relaxation Response* (New York: Morrow, 1975).

24. Jeanne Deschner, *The Hitting Habit: Anger Control for Battering Couples* (New York: The Free Press, 1984), pp. 52–53.

25. E. L. Phillips, D. L. Fixsen, and M. M. Wolfe, *The Teaching-Family Handbook*, Rev. ed. (Lawrence: Bureau of Child Research, University of Kansas, 1974).

26. Edward W. Gondolf and David Russell, "The Case Against Anger Control Treatment for Batterers," *Response*, Vol. 9, No. 3 (1986), pp. 2–5.

27. Ibid., p. 4.

28. In his chapter on preparing Othello for the National Theater, Olivier writes:

> To create a character, I first visualize a painting. . . . It began to come.
>
> I was beginning to know how I should look: very strong. He should stand like a strong man stands, with a sort of ease, straight-backed, straight-necked, relaxed as a lion. . . .
>
> A walk . . . I needed a walk. I must relax my feet. Get the right balance, not too taut, not too loose. . . . It wasn't working. . . . I took off my shoes and then my socks. Barefooted, the movement came. . . .
>
> I felt that Othello spoke differently from any other character in Shakespeare: he speaks like a foreigner who's learnt the language too carefully. . . .
>
> The voice. I was sure that he had a deeper voice than mine. Bass, a bass part, a sound that should be dark violet—velvet stuff. . . .
>
> The voice was of great importance. I began to work on it every day. I had to lower it, and slowly I surely did.

Sir Laurence Olivier, *On Acting* (London: George Weidenfeld & Nicholson Limited, 1986), pp. 105–106.

29. For example, liberal Protestant Adolf Harnack, in *What Is Christianity?* (New York: Harper and Brothers, Paperback, 1957), pp. 248–251, criticized the Roman Catholic tradition for corrupting the faith with Roman legalism.

6. The Molested

1. Estimates that one girl in four has suffered molestation derive from an early 1969 study of child sexual abuse by the Children's Division of the American Human Association, studies at the Kinsey Institute, Indiana University, and more recent reports by the clinician Dr. Henry Giarretto, Santa Clara County, California.

2. For one such study, see David Finkelhor, *Child Sexual Abuse: New Theory and Research* (New York: Macmillan, Free Press, 1984). Finkelhor reports that 19 percent of college women and 9 percent of college men (in six New England colleges) suffered sexual abuse as children.

3. The Human Association study reports the finding, which Finkelhor confirms, that 75 percent of the victims knew their abuser. See David Finkelhor, "A Survey of Sexual Abuse in the Population at Large," Department of Sociology, University of New Hampshire, NIMH Grants, T 32–MH15161 and R 01–MH30939, currently published in Finkelhor, *Child Sexual Abuse*, for further data in this paragraph and the following.

4. Charlotte Vale Allen, *Daddy's Girl* (New York: Wyndham Books, 1980).

5. See Sandra Butler, *Conspiracy of Silence, the Trauma of Incest* (Volcano, CA: Volcano Press, 1978), pp. 3–7 for details on the scope of incest.

6. For the following case and excellent comment, see Alayne Yates, M.D., "Children Eroticized by Incest," *American Journal of Psychiatry*, 139:4, (April 1982), pp. 482–485.

7. The quotations come from a transcript of Dr. Yates's videotaped interview with the foster mother and the two girls, by permission, Dr. Alayne Yates, Chief of Child Psychiatry, The University of Arizona, Health Sciences Center, Tucson, Arizona.

8. Yates, "Children Eroticized. . . '" p. 482.

9. Ibid.

10. Charlotte Vale Allen, *Daddy's Girl*, p. 58.

11. See Allen, ibid., pp. 58–60, for the ensuing dialogue.

12. Ibid., p. 60.

13. Ibid., p. 49.

14. Ibid., pp. 97–98.

15. Susan Forward and Craig Buck, *Betrayal of Innocence: Incest and Its Devastation* (Los Angeles: J. B. Tarcher, 1978), p. 62.

16. Dennis L. Bull, Ph.D., pamphlet of the Recovery Association, P.O. Box 821543, Dallas, TX 75382–1453.

17. Roland Summit, M.D., "Typical Characteristics of Father-Daughter Incest," unpublished paper, p. 25. Reprint requests to author, Head Physician, Community Consultation Service, Harbor-UCLA Medical Center, 1000 West Carson, Torrance, CA 90509.

18. Bull, pamphlet.

19. Butler, *Conspiracy of Silence*, p. 86.

20. Ibid., case of "Ingrid," pp. 149–155.

21. Allen, *Daddy's Girl*, p. 100.

22. Ernest Kurst, Ph.D., "Shame and Guilt: Characteristics of the Dependency Cycle," *Professional Education*, No. 7 (Center City, MN: Hazelden Foundation, 1981), p. 8.

23. Jacob and Wilhelm Grimm, "The Boy Who Left Home to Find Out About the Shivers," in *Grimm's Tales for Young and Old*, Tr. Ralph Manheim (Garden City, NY: Doubleday, 1977), pp. 12–19.

24. The Grimm brothers' story illumines here individuals who seem to have moved beyond the pale of ordinary human sensibility. The story aptly reveals institutional practices that seem affectless and unresponsive. See comments on the routine salvaging of organs in the chapter on organ transplants.

25. For extended discussion of some of the arguments for the *tabu* against incest, see Forward and Buck, *Betrayal of Innocence*.

26. Butler, *Conspiracy of Silence*, p. 60.

27. Summit, "Typical Characteristics . . . '" p. 25.

28. Butler, *Conspiracy of Silence*, pp. 133 and 140.

29. Ibid., p. 91.

30. Jan Varboe, "Wednesday's Child," *Texas Monthly*, August 1988, pp. 87ff.; Skip Hollandsworth, "The Uncertain Fate of Wednesday's Children," *D Magazine*, August 1988, pp. 45ff; Lisa Belkin, "Adoptive Parents Ask States for Help with Abused Young," *The New York Times*, August 22, 1988.

31. Henry Giarretto, Ph.D. "A Comprehensive Child Sexual Abuse Treatment Program," in *Sexually Abused Children and Their Families*, Patricia B. Mrazek and C. H. Kempe, eds. (Oxford: Pergamon Press, 1981).

32. Ibid., pp. 3–8.

33. Ibid.

34. Maggie Scarf's *Unfinished Business* (New York: Ballantine Books, 1980) at once describes the long reach of the past into the present and future of the depressed patient and the continuing task of renewal which the patient faces who would break the grip of that past.

7. The Aged

1. Ronald Blythe, *The View in Winter* (New York: Harcourt Brace Jovanovich, 1979), p. 8.

2. Ibid., p. 73.

3. Philip E. Slater, *The Pursuit of Loneliness* (Boston: Beacon Press, 1970), pp. 19 ff.

4. Blythe, *View in Winter*, p. 104.

5. Mr. Ahart, Director of Human Resources, testified before the House Select Committee on Aging, Feb. 22, 1978, 2nd Session, 95th Congress, that 25 percent of the elderly residents of total institutions were "misclassified" in that setting.

6. See "Communities for the Elderly," *Consumer Reports*, February 1990, for this quotation, p. 126, and for the following details in this paragraph, pp. 126–127.

7. Blythe, *View in Winter*, pp. 22–23.

8. John Yoder, *The Politics of Jesus* (Grand Rapids: Wm. B. Eerdmans, 1972), p. 174.

9. Ibid.

10. David Gutman, "The Premature Gerontocracy: Themes of Aging and Death in the Youth Culture," in *Death in American Experience*, Arien Mack, ed. (New York: Schocken Books, 1973).

11. As already indicated, caregivers need not only the virtue of love or benevolence associated with the role of giving in human life, but also humility, associated with the role of receiving. Caregivers need the virtue of humility as an antidote to their arrogance of power. They receive as well as give in the professional exchange.

12. For a study of the Benedictines, see Blythe's chapter on the "Prayer Route," in *View in Winter*, pp. 235–267.

13. The gerontologist Robert Butler has emphasized the importance for the elderly of life review. Workers in the hospice movement have adopted these techniques in their work with the dying.

14. Erik Erikson, *Identity, Youth and Crisis* (New York: W. W. Norton, 1968), pp. 139–140.

15. Ibid.

16. Ibid.

17. See May, *The Physician's Covenant*, Ch. 5, for a discussion of the virtues of nonchalance and courtesy as they bear on professional performance.

18. William Butler Yeats, *The Collected Poems of William Butler Yeats* (New York: Macmillan, 1976), p. 291.

8. Total Institutions

1. For a discussion of death as a "Hider-Goddess," see Edgar Herzog, *Psyche and Death, Archaic Myths and Modern Dreams in Analytical Psychology* (London: Hodder and Stroughton, 1966). Hermann Güntert's language studies of the Indo-Germanic (and pre-Indo-Germanic) period lead Herzog to state (p. 39) that a "mysterious hiding and shrouding has been experienced as the first essential character-trait of the numinous, hidden power of death in early times."

2. Erich Newmann, *The Origins and History of Consciousness* (Princeton, NJ:

Princeton University Press, First Princeton/Bollingen Paperback Printing, 1970). For further explorations of death as devourer, see Richard and Eva Blum, *Health and Healing in Rural Greece* (Stanford, CA: Stanford University Press, 1965), p. 129, and Herzog, *Psyche and Death*, Ch. 4, "The Death Demon as Dog and Wolf."

3. David J. Rothman, *The Discovery of the Asylum* (Boston: Little, Brown and Co., 1971), p. 95.

4. Ibid.

5. Erving Goffman, *Asylums* (Garden City, NY: Anchor Books, 1961), p. xiii.

6. Ibid., p. 14.

7. Ibid., p. 36.

8. Philip Elliot Slater, *The Pursuit of Loneliness* (Boston: Beacon Press, 1976), pp. 21–23.

9. Terry Colman, *Going to America* (New York: Random House, 1972), p. 216.

10. Michel Foucault, *Madness and Civilization* (New York: Random House, Vintage Books, 1973), p. 68.

11. Ibid., p. 7.

12. Ibid., p. 6.

13. See William F. May, *A Catalogue of Sins* (New York: Holt, Rinehart, and Winston, 1967), Ch. 6, for a fuller treatment of the sin of neglect.

14. Leo Strauss, *The Political Philosophy of Hobbes* (Oxford: The Clarendon Press, 1936), p. 9.

15. Ibid., p. 11.

16. The now-deceased Professor Arthur C. McGill of Harvard Divinity School offered the best examination of this topic in an as yet unpublished paper on "Identity and Death," in the care of the literary executor of his estate, Professor David Cain, Mary Washington College.

9. Alcoholics Anonymous

1. E. Kurtz, *Not-God: A History of Alcoholics Anonymous* (Center City, MN: Hazelden, 1979), p. 29.

2. *Alcoholics Anonymous* (New York: Alcoholics Anonymous World Services, Inc., 1976), p. 171.

3. *The Self-Help Sourcebook*, 1988, St. Claves Riverside Medical Center, Danville, NJ 07834.

4. Patricia Leigh Brown, "Troubled Millions Heed Call of Self Help Groups," *The New York Times*, July 16, 1988, pp. 1, 7.

5. The structural elements of law and story which shape AA reflect the polarities that have long determined the major Western religious traditions. The *halacha* (the law) and the *agada* (the narrative stories) constitute the two poles of Judaism (see Abraham Heschel, *God in Search of Man* [New York: The Jewish Publication Society, 1956], ch. 33). The Christian scriptures and later Christianity follow the same pattern, including both the law but also the gospel, the good news, the saving narrative of Jesus' birth, passion, death, and resurrection. In all cases, stories help provide the clarifying context that makes sense of the basic imperatives.

6. Nan Robertson, *Getting Better; Inside Alcoholics Anonymous* (New York: William Morrow and Company, 1988), p. 34.

7. Kurtz, *Not-God*, p. 197.

8. Ibid.

9. Robertson, *Getting Better*, p. 88

10. Ibid., p. 98.

11. Ibid., p. 115.
12. Ibid.
13. Ibid.
14. Ibid., p. 98.
15. "Elpenor," "A Drunkard's Progress," *Harper's* Vol. 273, October 1986, p. 44.
16. Karl Menninger, *Man Against Himself* (New York: Harcourt, Brace, 1938), pp. 149–154.
17. Robertson, *Getting Better*, Ch. 6.
18. Alcoholics Anonymous, Ch. 4.
19. The Twelve Steps appear on pp. 59–60 of *Alcoholics Anonymous*, receiving their basic exposition in chapters 5–7 of that volume. Subsequent quotations from the Twelve Steps will simply refer to the Step by number and not to the page number in the volume.
20. G. Van der Leeuw, *Religion in Essence and Manifestation*, Vol. I, p. 48.
21. "Elpenor," "A Drunkard's Progress," p. 45.
22. *Alcoholics Anonymous*, p. 59.
23. Karl Menninger, *Man Against Himself*, Part III.
24. *Alcoholics Anonymous*, p. 46.
25. Ibid., p. 45.
26. Ibid., pp. xxvi–xxvii.
27. Ibid., pp. 59, 63.
28. Harry M. Tiebout, "Surrender vs. Compliance Therapy," reprinted as a pamphlet by *Hazelden Educational Materials*, Box 176, Center City, MN 55012, with permission of the *Quarterly Journal of Alcohol Studies*, Vol. 14 (1953), pp. 58–68.
29. Ernest Kurtz, *Shame and Guilt: Characteristics of the Dependency Cycle*, Vol. 7 in series on Professional Education (Center City, MN: Hazelden Foundation, 1981), p. 19.
30. Ibid., p. 8.
31. Ibid., pp. 6–9.
32. *Alcoholics Anonymous* carries the Twelve Traditions in short form, p. 564, and in long form, pp. 565–568. All subsequent references to the Twelve Traditions will cite the number of the tradition rather than the page number in the volume.
33. See Kurtz, *Not-God*, p. 197, for an exploration of strength in weakness.
34. Cited by Robertson, *Getting Better*, p. 73.
35. Kurtz, *Not-God*, p. 123.
36. See Harry M. Tiebout, M.D., "The Role of Psychiatry in the Field of Alcoholism," distributed by the National Council on Alcoholism, Inc., 733 Third Ave., New York, NY 10017. For a brief account of Dr. Jellinek's views in *The Disease Concept of Alcoholism* (New Haven, CT: College and University Press, 1960), consult Robertson, *Getting Better*, pp. 190–192, 196–197.
37. "Elpenor," "A Drunkard's Progress," p. 46.
38. *Alcoholics Anonymous*, p. 39. Bill Wilson points to a man still trapped in the illusion that knowledge will solve his problem: Fred was positive that "self-knowledge would fix it." Ibid., p. 40.
39. Ibid., p. 43.
40. Cited by Robertson, *Getting Better*, p. 125.
41. *Alcoholics Anonymous*, p. 180.
42. Eventually the American Public Health Association gave AA the Lasker Award and cited it for "creating an ever expanding chain reaction of liberation, with patients welded together by bonds of common suffering, common

understanding. . ." (Robertson, *Getting Better*, p. 91). It foresaw (in 1951) that this new therapy would have a "vast potential for the myriad other ills of humankind." In fact, AA has provided a prototype for the myriad support groups to which millions of sufferers have turned since the inception of AA, not necessarily to eliminate problems but to face them humanly.

10. Organ Donations

1. Umehara Takeshi, "A Buddhist Approach to Organ Transplants," *Japan Echo*, Vol. 16, Number 4, 1989.

2. "A Definition of Irreversible Coma," *Journal of the American Medical Association* 205:337–40, 1968.

3. The Hastings Center (then called The Institute of Society, Ethics and the Life Sciences) Task Force on Death and Dying, "Refinements in Criteria for the Determination of Death," *Journal of the American Medical Association*, 221 (1):48–53, July 3, 1972.

4. The UDDA states: "An individual who has sustained either 1) irreversible cessation of circulatory functions, or 2) irreversible cessation of all functions of the entire brain, including the brain stem is dead. A determination of death must be made in accordance with accepted medical standards." Cited in *Deciding to Forego Life-Sustaining Treatment; Ethical, Medical and Legal Issues in Treatment Decisions*, the President's Commission for the Study of Ethical Problems in Medicine and Biomedical and Behavioral Research, March 1983, pp. 9–10.

5. George Simenon, *Maigret and the Headless Corpse*, E. Ellen-Bogen, trans. (New York: Harcourt, Brace, and World, 1967), p. 147.

6. "Organ Donation, Approach to Next of Kin," UK Transplant Coordinator Association, obtained from Oxford office, Great Britain.

7. UNOS, 3001 Hungary Spring Road, P. O. Box 2810, Richmond, Virginia 23228.

8. Joel Feinberg, *Offense to Others*, Vol. II of *The Moral Limits of the Criminal Law* (New York: Oxford University Press, 1985), p. 80.

9. Ibid., p. 82.

10. Robert W. Boven conducted the survey for the *International Organ and Tissue Retrieval Directory* (5th Edition, 1980).

11. St. Augustine, *Nicene and Post-Nicene Fathers*, 1st Series, Vol. III, ed. by Philip Schaff, tr. by H. Browne (Grand Rapids: William B. Eerdmans, 1956).

12. D. Alan Shewman, "Anencephaly: Selected Medical Aspects," *Hastings Center Report*, October/November 1988, Vol. 18, No. 5, pp. 11–18.

13. Ibid., p. 17.

14. Alexander Capron, "Anencephalic Donors: Separate the Dead from the Dying," *Hastings Center Report*, February 1987, Vol. 17, No. 1, p. 8.

15. Ibid.

16. Gilbert Meilaender, "Case Studies: The Anencephalic Newborn as Donor," *Hastings Center Report*, April 1986, Vol. 16, No. 2, p. 23.

17. John A. Robertson, author of "Rights, Symbolism, and Public Policy in Fetal Tissue Transplants," *Hastings Center Report*, December 1988, Vol. 18, No. 5, p. 5, derives his data on abortions from Stanley K. Henshaw et al., "A Portrait of American Women Who Obtain Abortions," *Family Planning Perspectives*, 17:2 (1985), 90–96, and Kevin Lafferty, statement to the Fetal Tissue Transplantation Research Panel, National Institutes of Health, September 15, 1988.

18. *Report of the Human Fetal Tissue Transplantation Research Panel*, Advisory to the Director of the National Institutes of Health, December 1988, Vol. II, p. E 1.

19. Kathleen Nolan, "Genug ist Genug: A Fetus is Not a Kidney," *Hastings Center Report*, December 1988, Vol. 18, No. 6, p. 14.

20. James Burtchaell, "Case Study: University Policy on Experimental Use of Aborted Fetal Tissue," *IRB: A Review of Human Subjects Research*, 10:4 (July/August 1988), pp. 7–11.

21. Dr. Carl Kjellstrand presented his paper "Limited Resources in the Developed World—Have Doctors Satisfied Their Duty to Justice?" at the International Congress on Ethics, Justice, and Commerce in Transplantation: A Global Issue, hosted by Health and Welfare Canada and the Transplantation Society, August 20–24, 1989, Ottawa, Canada. It is slated for publication in the proceedings of the Congress.

22. James F. Childress, "Organ Transplants: Policies, Practices, and Principles," a paper originally presented at the Woodrow Wilson Center, Washington, D.C., portions of which appear under the title "Ethical Criteria for Procuring and Distributing Organs for Transplantation" in *Journal of Health Politics, Policy and Law*, Vol. 14, No. 1 (Spring 1989), pp. 102–110.

23. James F. Childress, "Who Shall Live When Not All Can Live?" *Soundings: An Interdisciplinary Journal*, Vol. 53, No. 4 (Winter 1970), pp. 339–355.

24. See James F. Childress, "Ethical Criteria for Procuring and Distributing Organs for Transplantation," pp. 102–110, and "Some Moral Connections Between Organ Procurement and Organ Distribution," *Journal of Contemporary Health Law and Policy*, Vol. 3, 1987, pp. 95–110.

25. Meilaender, "Case Studies. . . .'" p. 23.

Postscript

1. Arthur C. McGill, *Death and Life: An American Theology*, Charles A. Wilson and Per M. Anderson, eds. (Philadelphia: Fortress Press, 1987), p. 94.

2. Ibid.

3. Ibid.

4. Ibid., p. 95.

5. Ibid., p. 85.

6. See May, *The Physician's Covenant*, chapters 1 and 2, for an extended treatment of the two images of the parent and the fighter as ways of interpreting the physician's role. See also Arthur C. McGill, *Death and Life: An American Theology*, published posthumously.

7. The unorthodox Eastern Orthodox theologians Vladimir Soloviov and Nicholas Berdyaev and the redoubtable Protestant theologian Karl Barth recognized the driving force of death's denial at work in building civilizations and careers alike. See Berdyaev's *The Destiny of Man* (London: Geoffrey Bles: The Centenary Press, 1937), pp. 236, 317–337, and Barth's *Church Dogmatics*, Vol. IV, Pt. 2 (Edinburgh: T & T Clark, 1958), pp. 467–483. Ernest Becker, in his searching *The Denial of Death* (New York: The Free Press, 1973), chapters 2 and 4, has more recently sounded the same theme. See also William F. May, *Dread Before Death and Revolt Against Death: A Study of Heidegger and Camus*, Ph.D. dissertation, Yale University, 1961, and "The Sacral Power of Death in Contemporary Experience" in *Perspectives on Death*, Liston O. Mills, ed. (Nashville: Abingdon Press, 1969), pp. 168–196.

WILLIAM F. MAY is Cary M. Maguire
Professor of Ethics at Southern Methodist
University and author of *A Catalogue of Sins*
and *The Physician's Covenant: Images of the
Healer in Medical Ethics*.